Mapo tofu 麻婆豆腐

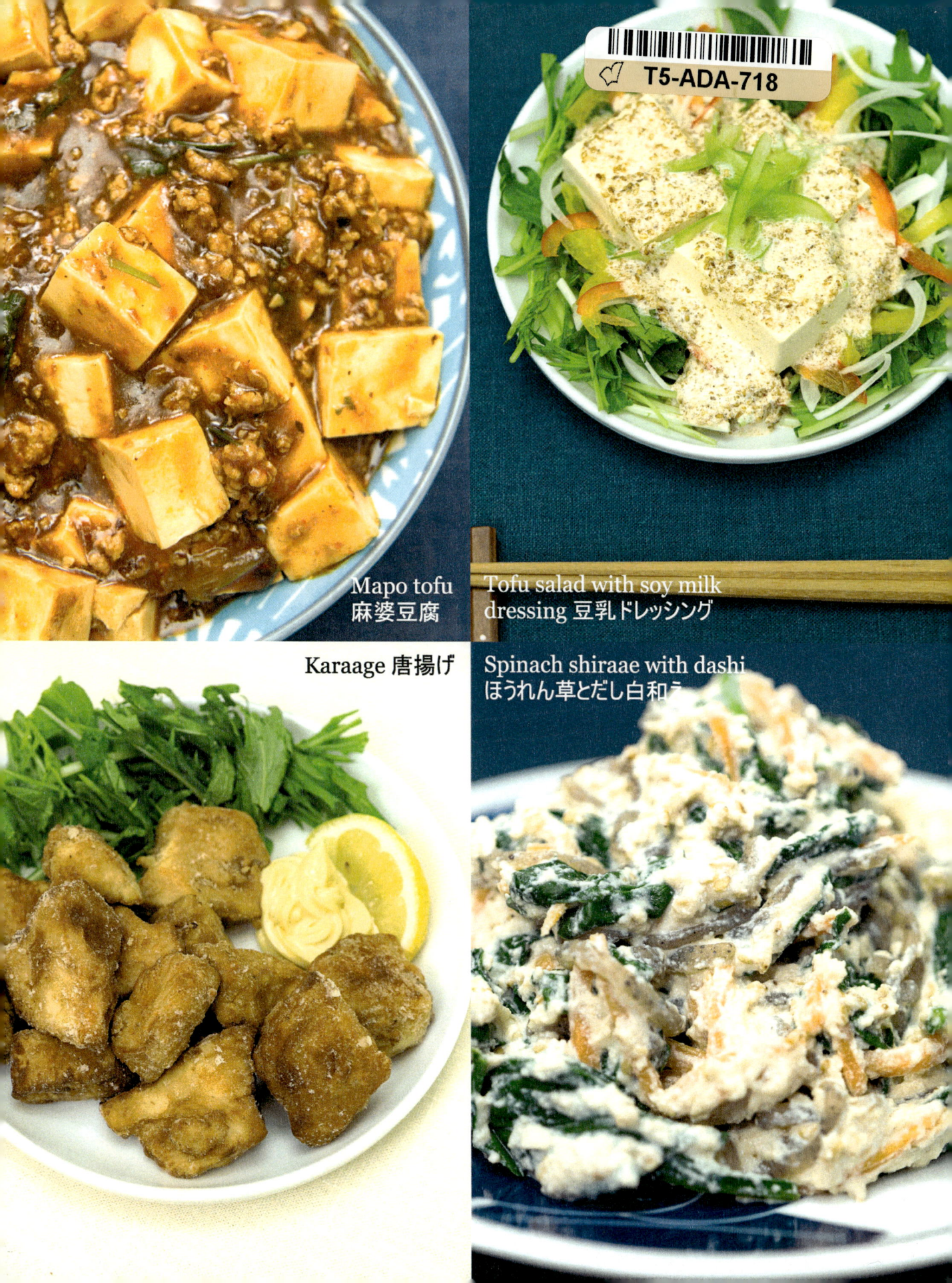

Tofu salad with soy milk dressing 豆乳ドレッシング

Karaage 唐揚げ

Spinach shiraae with dashi ほうれん草とだし白和え

Contents

Introduction P. 6

What's tofu and how's it made? P. 9
  Common types of tofu P. 10
  Working with tofu P. 12

Before you start P. 14
  Japanese Pantry P. 16

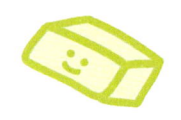

Dashi
- ●●● Konbu dashi 昆布だし P. 20
- ●● Ichiban and niban dashi だし P. 22
- ●● Sansho tsukudani 山椒佃煮 P. 24

Cold tofu dishes

Hiyayakko 冷奴 P. 26
- ● Negishio, umekatsuo, shisoginger ネギ塩、梅かつお、しそと生姜 P. 28
- ● Yuzukosho and sansho tsukudani 柚子胡椒と山椒佃煮 P. 29
- ●●● Umejiso 梅干しとしそ P. 30
- ●● Shiso, miso and tomato しそと味噌とトマト P.31
- ● Natto okra 納豆オクラ
- ●●● Negishiokoji ねぎ塩麹 P. 33

Tofu Salads 豆腐サラダ
- ●●● Tofu salad with sesame vinaigrette 胡麻ドレッシング P. 36
- ●● Tofu salad with gomadare ごまだれ P. 38
- ●● Tofu salad with soy milk dressing 豆乳ドレッシング P. 40

Shiraae 白和え
- ●●● Spinach shiraae ほうれん草白和え P. 44
- ●● Spinach shiraae with dashi ほうれん草とだし白和え P. 46
- ●●● Green bean shiraae インゲン白和え P. 48
- ●●● Asparagus shiraae アスパラ白和え P. 49

● *vegan* ● *vegetarian* ● *meat-free* ● *dairy-free* ● *gluten-free*

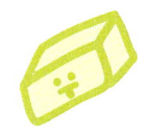

Warm tofu dishes P. 50
- ●●● Miso dengaku 味噌田楽 P. 52
- ●● Ankakedoufu あんかけ豆腐 P. 54
- ●● Kinoko ankakedoufu きのこあんかけ豆腐 P. 56
- ●● Karaage 唐揚げ P. 58
- ●●● Atsuage 厚揚げ P. 60
- ●●● Teriyaki atsuage 照り焼き厚揚げ P. 62
- ●●● Tofu steaks with kabayaki sauce 豆腐蒲焼ステーキ P. 64
- ●●● Tofu steaks with nira Dressing ニラドレッシング P. 66
- ● Tofu tosayaki 豆腐土佐焼 P. 70
- ● Tsukune つくね P. 72

Main dishes P. 74
- ●●● Iridoufu 煎り豆腐 P. 76
- ● Mapo-tofu 麻婆豆腐 P. 78
- ●● Chikuzenni 筑前煮 P. 80
- ●● Tofu tounyuu nabe 豆腐豆乳鍋 P.83
- ●●●● Momiji oroshi 紅葉おろし P. 86
- ●● Lemon ponzu レモンポン酢 P. 87
- ●●● Nirajouyu ニラ醤油 P. 89
- Tofu hamburger 豆腐ハンバーグ P. 90
- ● Nikudoufu 肉豆腐 P. 92
- ●● Tofu gyoza 豆腐餃子 P. 94

● *vegan* ● *vegetarian* ● *meat-free* ● *dairy-free* ● *gluten-free*

Next Steps P. 97

About the author P. 99

Acknowledgements P. 100

Resources P. 101

Frequently Asked Questions P. 102

Introduction

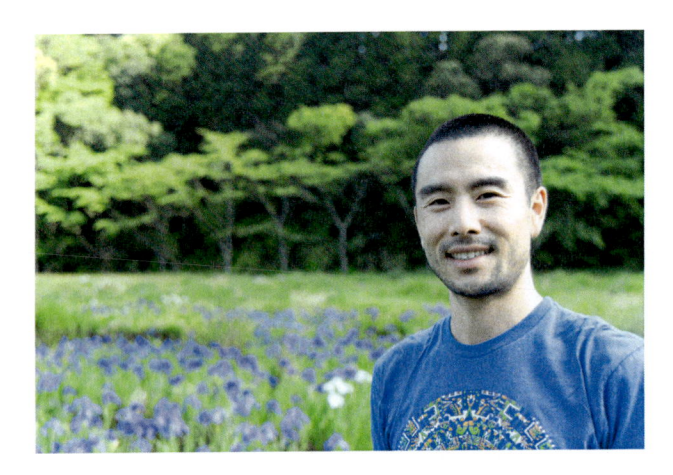

Hi! I'm Pat Tokuyama. I've been eating tofu for as long as I can remember. But it wasn't until I was in my 20s that the tofu love bug bit me. (Ouch!)

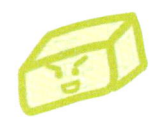

My eating experiences at Tofu Ryouri (豆腐料理) specialty restaurants in Japan were transformational.

An entire meal with multiple courses centered around tofu and soy? Mind blown!

Taste buds too! Whenever I visit Japan, I always make a point to eat at one.

I'm always amazed at how an entire meal could be so varied and delicious, despite serving nothing but multiple courses of tofu and soy-based dishes.

My favorites tend to be the yuba (soy milk skin), dengaku (sweet savory miso glaze), yudofu (tofu cooked in dashi broth), and of course the desserts!

These restaurant menus are not only healthy and delicious, but also very labor intensive.

But don't worry, I'm not trying to recreate those experiences.

At least not yet.

For now, we're sticking to simple recipes in this book.

These restaurant experiences are just one part of the inspiration for this book.

So what else caused me to write this book? Why tofu?

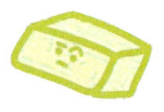

Start Here

Who is Tofu Ryouri for ?
This book may be for you if...
- you want to get started cooking Japanese food, but aren't sure how
- you have some experience cooking Japanese food, but not much with tofu
- you've been to Japan and want to recreate authentic Japanese flavors at home
- you're curious about cooking and/or cooking with tofu
- you like tofu but are tired of the same old recipes and want something new
- you want to improve your cooking skills
- you consider yourself a foodie
- you enjoy learning and trying new things
- you like a challenge
- you want to eat more sustainably
- you want to eat healthier, tasty foods that are easy to prepare

Who Tofu Ryouri is NOT for -
This book may not be for you if...
- you don't like tofu or soy based foods
- you don't like Japanese foods or flavors
- you don't like cooking
- you feel like you have enough recipes and cookbooks
- you aren't looking to eat healthier
- you aren't interested in learning or stepping out of your comfort zone
- you enjoy cooking without recipes
- you enjoy meat-centric dishes

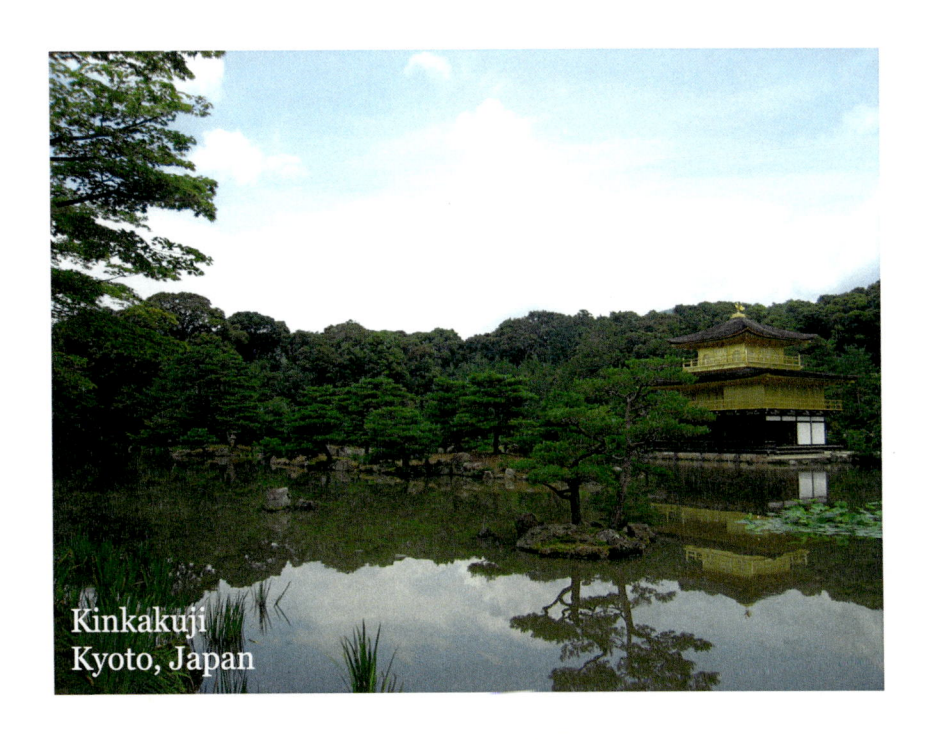

Kinkakuji
Kyoto, Japan

Your FREE BONUS

Your learning doesn't stop with this book! To say thank you, I wanted to provide some additional material 100% FREE!

Get your FREE bonus materials at www.alldayieat.com/bookbonus

Some of the FREE bonus materials include:
- a behind the scenes look at the creation of this book with photos and videos
- a behind the scenes look at my blog, recipe, and video creation process
- more delicious Japanese recipes and how-to videos
- 5-7 day Japanese cooking challenges
- exclusive access to the new online Tofu Ryouri Cooking Program
- and more!

Head over to www.alldayieat.com/bookbonus to get your FREE bonus materials now!

It's FREE!

Here's the story.

Back in August 2016, the afternoon before I was to leave on a surf trip to Costa Rica, I had just finished an epic surf session... I was getting out of the water and sprained my ankle.

Long story short, I couldn't walk for a little over a month. During that time, I had all this energy and couldn't participate in my usual surfing, running, and outdoor activities.

So I decided to start a food blog - All day I eat like a shark which was born in August of 2016.

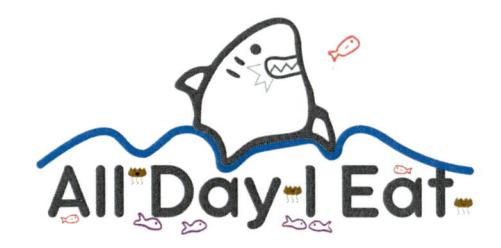

During this time, I also read a lot. A few of the books I read about food and nutrition made me realize I could really improve my diet. (see resources P. 101)

These books led me to change my perspectives on food, as well as, my eating habits.

The major changes I made were paying closer attention to the food I buy (e.g. organic, local and in season), cooking with fresh food (e.g. no more mixes, boxed, or premade foods), and significantly cutting back on meat.

I have an extensive family history of cancers, heart disease, as well as diabetes. While a long life may be in my genes, chronic disease is too.

Diet and lifestyle both play a significant role in your overall health.

And as a pharmacist, I know that a healthy lifestyle goes a long way in preventing chronic diseases, especially as I reach my golden years.

One of the ways I try to eat healthy is by cooking more Japanese food than I used to.

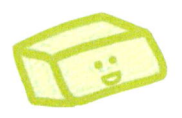

As I experienced firsthand, the power that books can have on one's life, I thought it might be time to step up and do something similar, in my own way, with a cookbook.

It didn't take long for me to decide on the topic for this Japanese cookbook.

As I mentioned before, some of my fondest travel memories include eating at tofu restaurants in Japan.

So I couldn't think of a better, more exciting way, than to inspire and guide you on a culinary journey through Japan with tofu!

Tofu ryouri (豆腐料理) literally translated means tofu cooking.

And I want this book to show you that cooking healthy Japanaese food isn't that difficult.

And that it can be especially delicious and fun, despite using one main ingredient – tofu.

Perhaps, you'll change your mind about tofu/Japanese cuisine after trying a few of the recipes or perhaps you won't.

The choice is yours!

Thank you for allowing me to serve you and I wish you the best in your tofu and non-tofu cooking adventures!

-pat

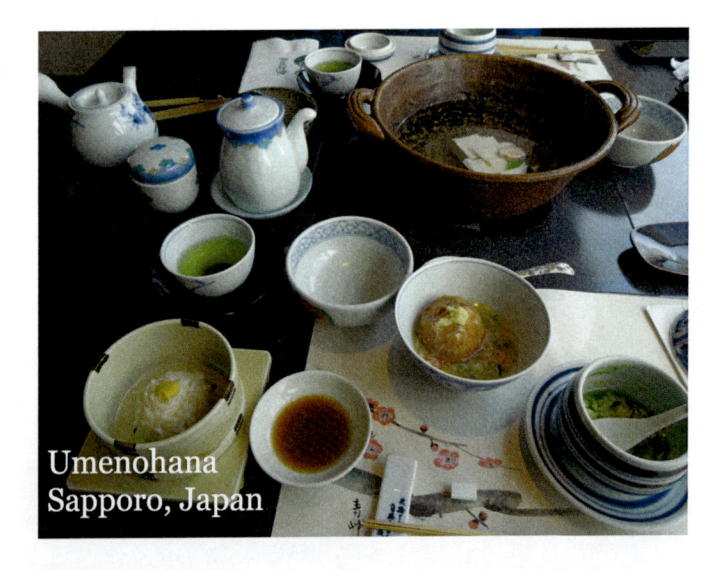

Umenohana
Sapporo, Japan

What's tofu and how's it made?

Tofu is also known as bean curd. Tofu is naturally gluten-free, low in calories, low in fat, and high in protein. It also contains a good amount of iron and calcium or magnesium, depending on the salts used to make it.

It's healthy, nutritious, easy to cook with, and even easier to eat. It doesn't have much of a strong flavor on its own, so it can be used in a wide variety of savory appetizers, main courses to baked goods and sweet desserts!

In its purest form, tofu consists of soy milk with added calcium or magnesium salts. Acids like glucono-delta-lactone can also be used.

Both salt and acid alter the proteins in soy milk, which causes curdling, or coagulation.

Once curdled, water can be pressed out to make a block of tofu; the more water that's removed, the firmer the tofu.

If you've never made it yourself, here's how I make it in 5 steps.

1. Dried soy beans (大豆 - daizu) are soaked in water (8+ hours) to be rehydrated.
2. Rehydrated beans are then pureed with water. This is called namago (生呉).
3. Once the namago is heated, the soy milk (豆乳 - tounyuu) and the pulp (おから - okara) can be separated.
4. To turn soy milk into tofu, a coagulant (にがり - nigari) is added to the milk. This causes the milk to curdle and naturally thicken up.
5. The curdled milk is then put in a mold and pressed to make a block of tofu!

I remember the first time I had fresh soy milk turn to tofu.

It was at an izakaya (居酒屋 - pub like restaurant for food/drink) and watching the soy milk turn into tofu was like magic!

First it was liquid and after adding the coagulant (it looked like salt), the liquid turned into a solid mass!

All it took was a few minutes and my life was forever changed!

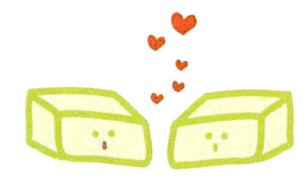

Common types of tofu

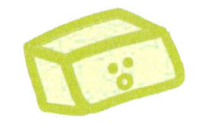

For the recipes in this book, we'll be using either firm or soft tofu.

Firm tofu is also known as momendofu (木綿豆腐 - 'Cotton' tofu). To make firm tofu, the coagulated soymilk is put into molds lined with a cloth and then pressed to remove excess water.

This results in a dense and firm tofu with a rough texture and more protein per bite. This makes it best for grilling, pan frying, simmering, or deep frying.

Soft tofu is less firm than firm tofu but not as soft as silken tofu. It's in the middle.

It's easy to work with and for many of the recipes in this book, interchangeable with firm tofu.

Soft tofu is my favorite since it's got a soft texture that's almost as soft as silken, but doesn't quite melt in your mouth.

Silken tofu is also known as kinugoshi (絹ごし豆腐) tofu. It has a very fine and smooth texture, think panna cotta - that isn't as sweet and jiggles.

Silken tofu is not as easy to work with as soft tofu, and may not be available unless you live near a tofu producer.

The good thing is that you can make it at home if you make soy milk!

You just need nigari! (see resources P. 101)

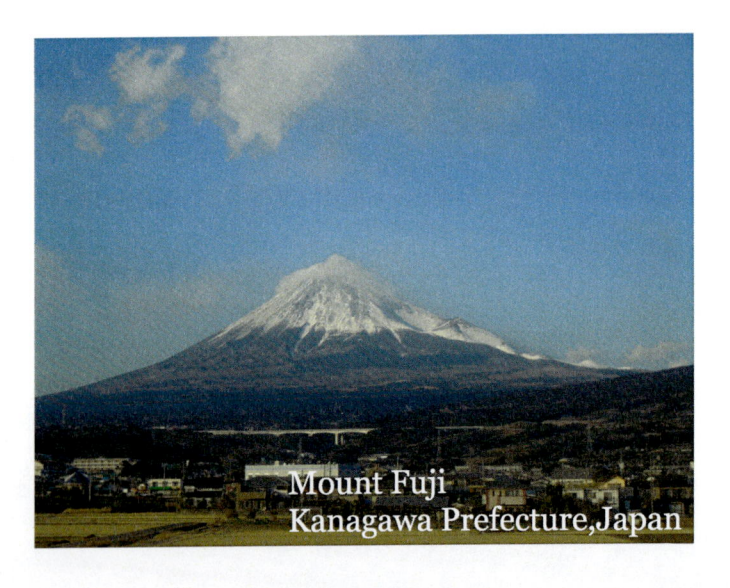

Mount Fuji
Kanagawa Prefecture, Japan

Soft tofu blocks

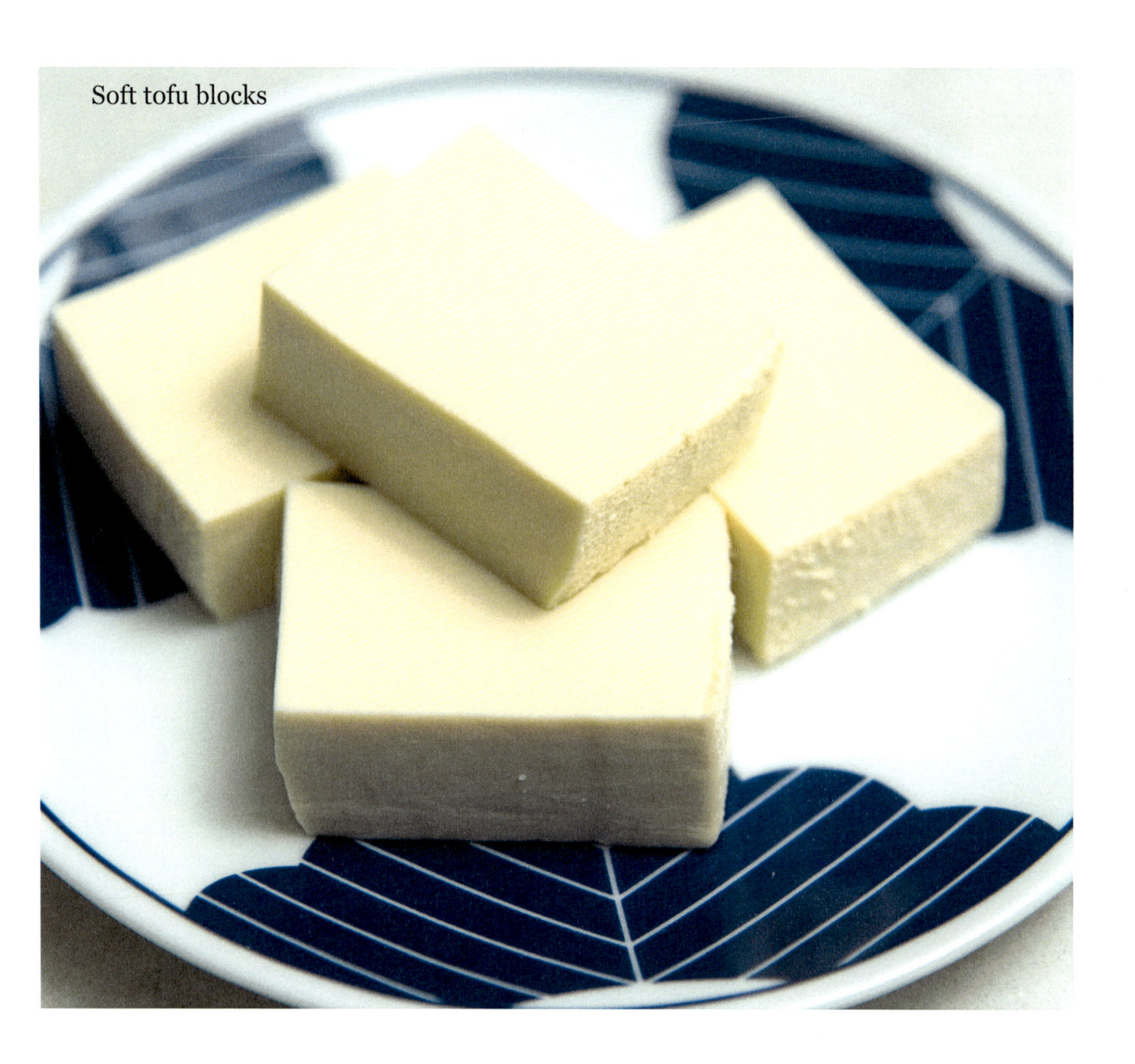

Working with tofu

The primary types of tofu I use in this book are soft tofu and firm tofu. One of the key steps in making these dishes a success is removing excess water from the tofu.

Tofu is over 80% water. So if not drained properly you'll end up with a diluted seasoning or sauce.

By removing excess water, you also concentrate the tofu flavor, umami, and improve the texture. If you're frying it, it'll reduce any splattering caused by water mixing with oil.

There are several ways you can remove excess water from tofu. Also referred to as mizuwokiru (水を切る), literally to cut the water.

Here are five ways to remove excess water (longest to shortest)
1. Cutting and allowing the water to leak out.
    Pro - no 'work' required, can be used for hot or cold dishes
    Con - requires plates/bowls, can make a mess (water), takes 60 minutes+

2. Placing a weight on top of the tofu. Use at least 5 pounds (2-3kg) and something to balance it, if necessary. Allow to sit 45 minutes to an hour. You'll also need a shallow plate or bowl to catch the water being squeezed out.
    Pro - good for cold dishes, takes less time than the above, need to plan ahead
    Con - requires plates/bowls, can make a mess (water), takes at least 45 minutes

3. Using a tofu pressing device, which presses on the tofu, squeezing out excess water.
    Pro - easy to use, can be done ahead of time, best for firm tofu, the longer you press it the more water will come out
    Con - larger blocks may not fit, takes at least 15-20 minutes

4. Using the stove with a pot of boiling water. You can boil the tofu for 3-5 minutes and then drain and pat dry. This method is most effective when the tofu is cut into blocks.
    Pro - quick with minimal prep, good for warm dishes, no need to plan
    Con - the tofu will be very hot and you need to not only let it cool, but also drain and pat dry once you can handle it, not good if you need cold tofu

5. Microwaving with a tea towel or paper towel for 2-3 minutes.
    Pro - quick with minimal prep, good for warm preparations, no need to plan
    Con - you have to use a paper towel or tea towel, which may stick to your soft tofu and cause it to break, not good if you need cold tofu, may get slightly deformed

Unpressed tofu left, pressed right

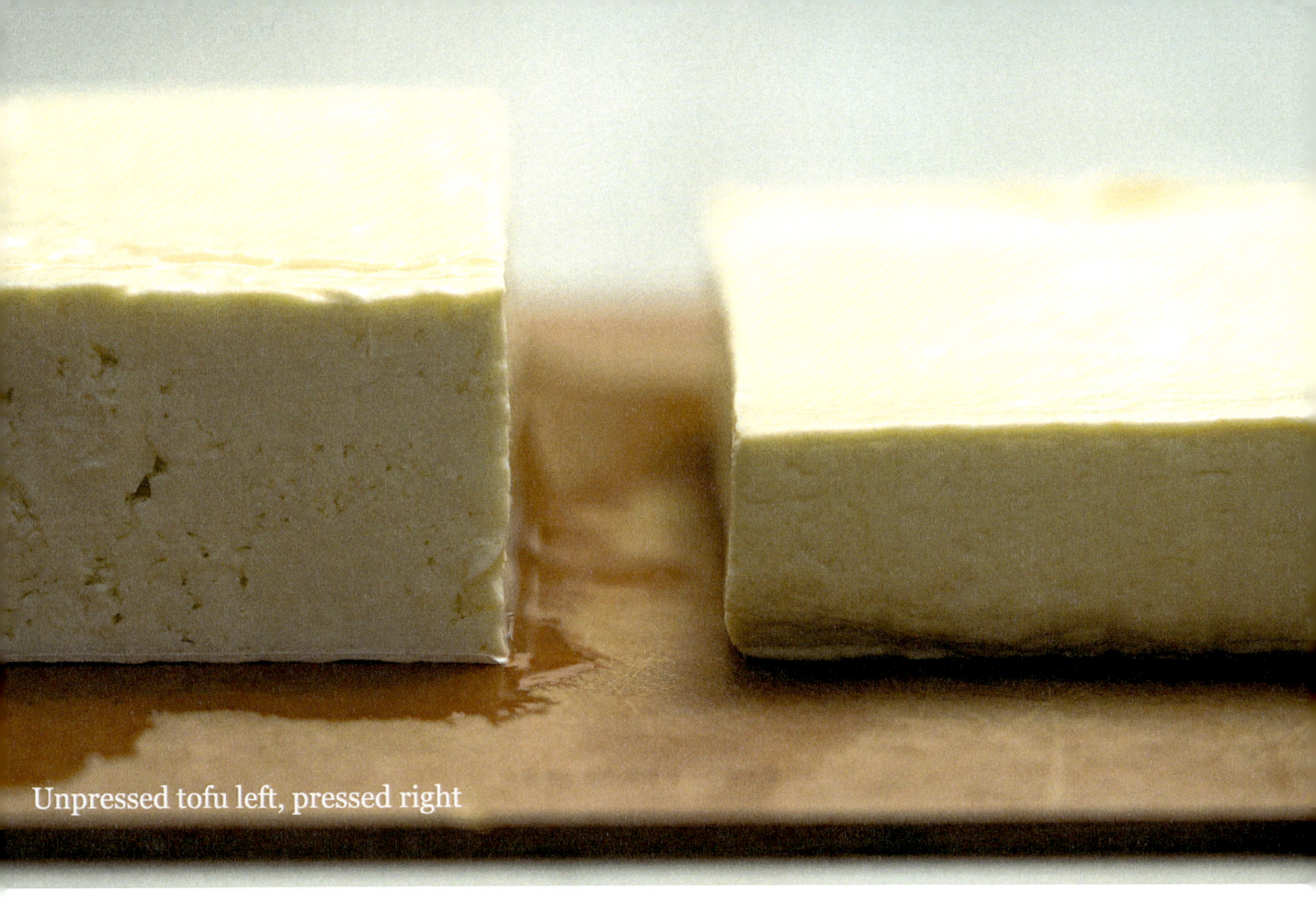

Important Note

Tofu blocks come in many different sizes. For the recipes in this book, one block of tofu is 14 oz.

For each recipe in this book, I've removed excess water **ahead of time**, unless microwaving or cooking on stove.

So make sure to follow one of the methods discussed previously to remove excess water from your tofu.

You can remove excess water for any tofu recipe.

This technique is not limited to Japanese cooking and will help to enhance the flavor and seasoning of any dish that calls for tofu!

Before you start...

Japanese food may seem exotic, but once you get a few basic recipes down, many of them have similar techniques.

The majority of the recipes in this book take less than 30 minutes start to finish, with some exceptions like gyoza requiring a little more time. I wanted to make your cooking experience as smooth as possible, by including dishes that were simple, with easy to access ingredients and taste great.

A good portion of Japanese recipes call for the same key ingredients- sake, mirin, soy sauce, dashi, and miso.

In the next few pages, we'll review these key ingredients and a few more that are used in this book. If you can't find these key ingredients at your market, they're available online. See resources P. 101 for additional information.

(left to right - sake, mirin, soy sauce, light soy sauce, rice vinegar, sesame oil)

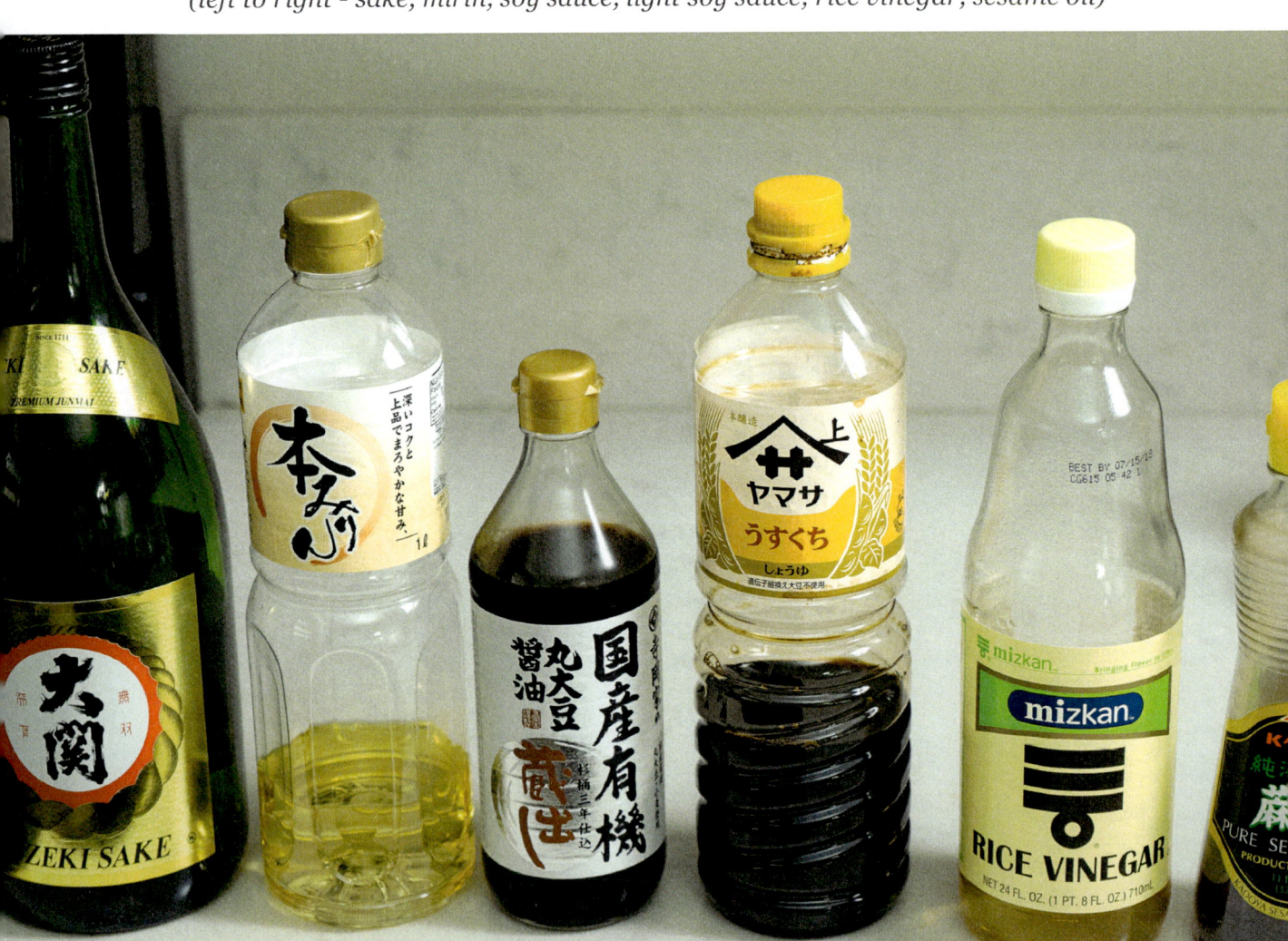

Konbu

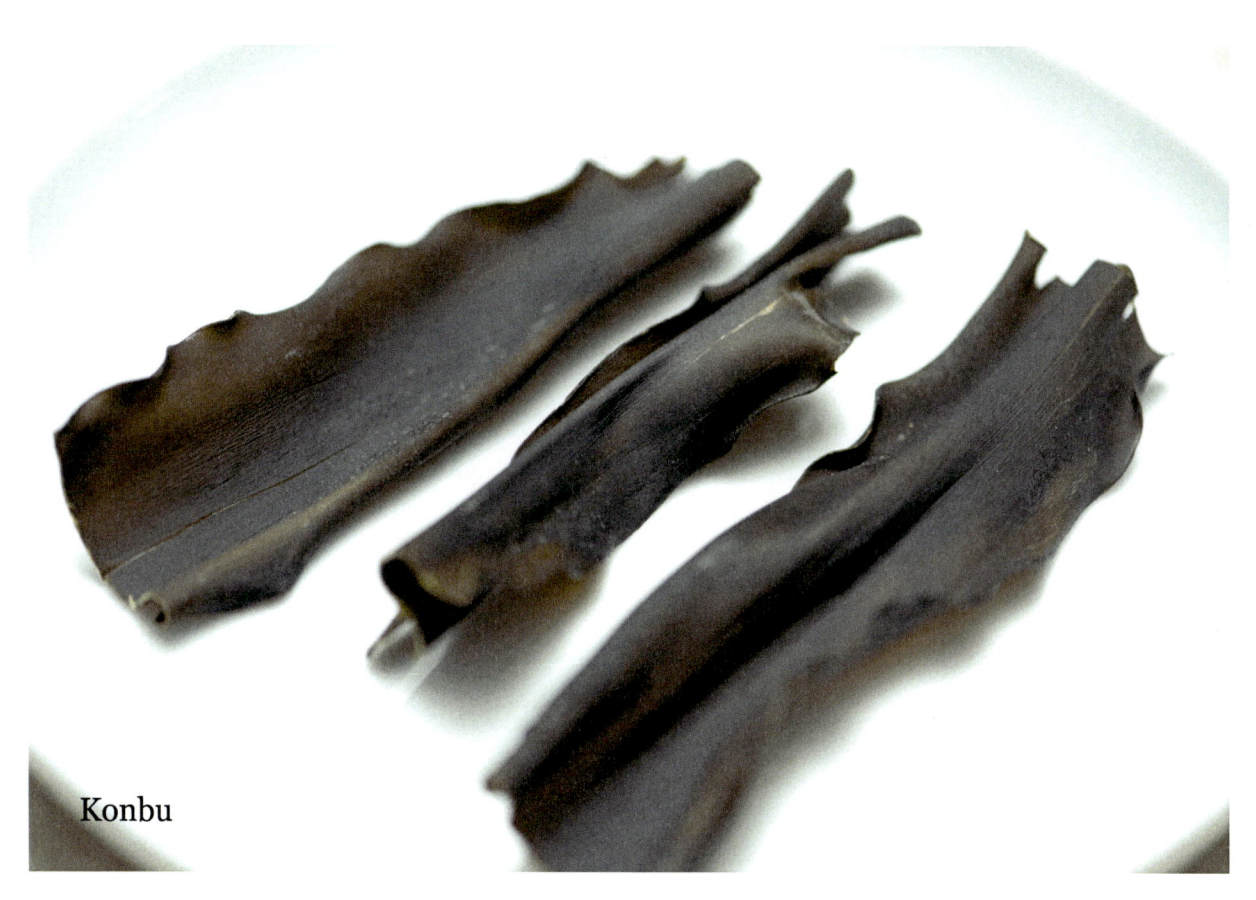

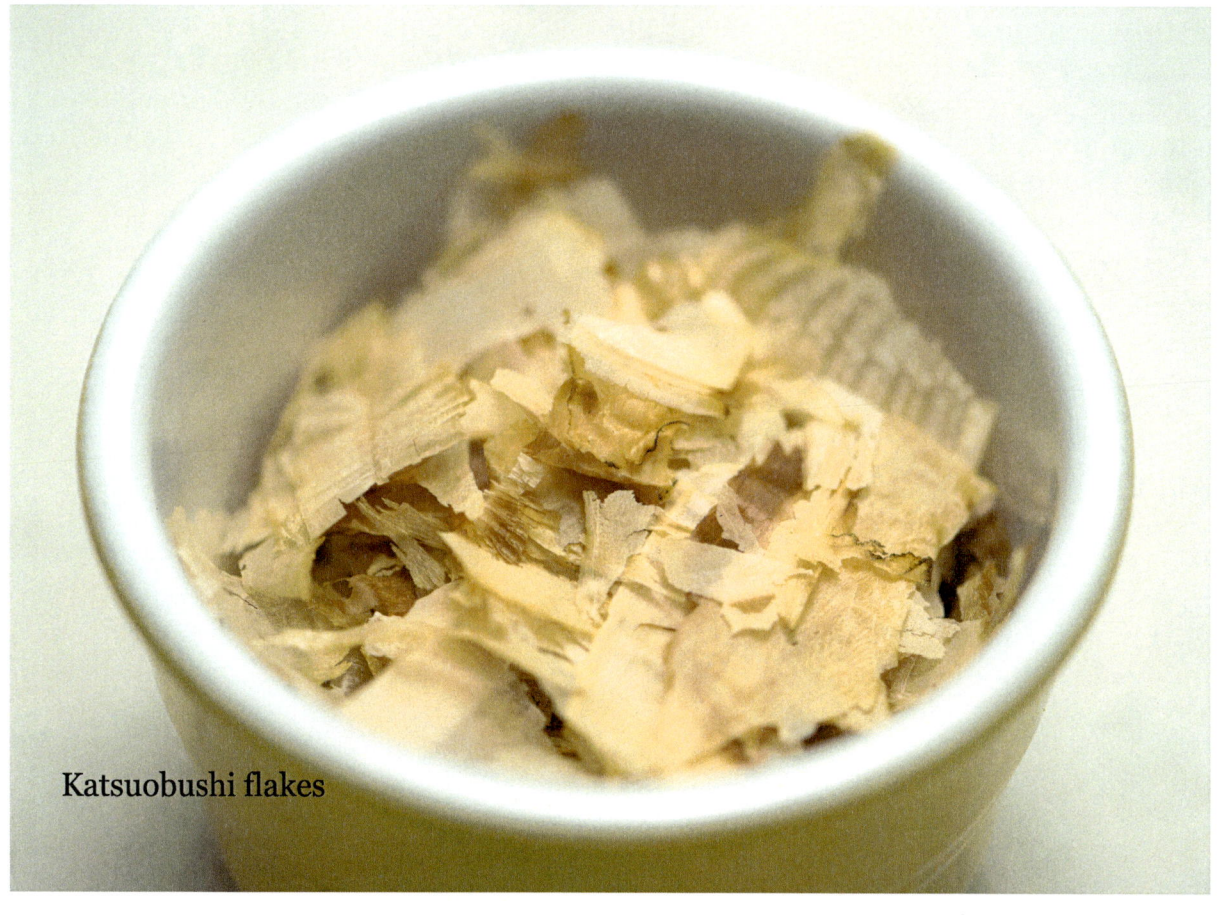

Katsuobushi flakes

Japanese Pantry

Sake お酒

Sake is basically rice and water that's been fermented with yeast. It has an alcohol content ranging from 15-20%. Sake has several effects on your food. It helps to tenderize meats and vegetables, enhance the natural flavors of your food, while decreasing any unpleasant odors or flavors.

Thanks to the fermentation process it has a natural sweetness and range of flavors from floral, fruity, herbaceous, and spiced among others. It's also packed with flavor enhancing amino acids like glutamic acid. Glutamic acid is one of many umami producing compounds.

Tip: I tend to avoid cooking sake because it has salt added to it, which isn't necessary. For cooking, you can use regular drinking sake and it doesn't need to be expensive.

Mirin 味醂

Mirin is made by fermenting steamed glutinous rice, kome-koji (米麴 - rice with mold koji – Aspergillus oryzae) and alcohol for several months. It's then pressed and filtered, which results in a sweet and slightly thick liquid. It has a mild sweet flavor and adds depth to foods you cook with it. Like sake, it contains amino acids (umami flavors) and also minimizes fishy, meaty flavors when used as a marinade.

Shoyu 醬油 (soy sauce)

Soy sauce is made from soy beans, wheat, salt and water. The recipes in this book call for two of the more common types.

Usukuchi shoyu (薄口醬油 - light soy sauce) and koikuchi shoyu (濃口醬油 - dark soy sauce).

Dark soy sauce is simply referred to as shoyu. This is your all-purpose soy sauce. It has about a 16% salt content. It's the most commonly used soy sauce in Japanese cooking.

Usukuchi shoyu on the other hand has a higher salt content (18-19%). Light soy sauce also has less of a strong flavor and a lighter color. These aspects help to enhance the natural color and flavor of the food it seasons.

Note - It's easy to get light soy sauce confused with low-sodium soy sauce. Remember that these are two completely different soy sauces. Low-sodium soy sauce is koikuchi soy sauce with less sodium. I do recommend using low sodium soy sauce when possible. I've found no significant difference in flavor and it also helps to limit salt intake.

Rice vinegar お酢

Osu (お酢 - rice vinegar) is a key ingredient for Japanese pickles. Japanese rice vinegar has a unique flavor which I find relatively mild. We'll use rice vinegar primarily for salad dressings here, but note it's also used to make sushi rice (or shari in sushi slang) and sauces like nanbanzuke and for gyoza!

Sesame oil 胡麻油

Gomaabura (胡麻油 - sesame oil) is a dark and fragrant oil used for a variety of dishes. I primarily use it for salads (dressings), stir frys or fried foods like karaage.

Katsuobushi 鰹節

Katsuobushi is available in blocks or preshaved flakes. The blocks are made by smoking, fermenting, and drying boiled or steamed skipjack tuna. The blocks eventually need to be shaved before use and you can do it yourself (if you want a work out) or buy them shaved and ready for use. This along with konbu forms the base dashi that you can use to make many Japanese dishes.

Konbu 昆布

Konbu is kelp which has been harvested from the ocean then dried in the sun. It's a very labor intensive process which is one of the reasons it can be one of the more expensive ingredients. However, note that there's nothing like it and it contains many naturally occurring umami compounds. These compounds are what gives certain dishes a unique and rich, delicate flavor.

Miso 味噌

Miso is made from steamed soy beans that have been mixed with salt, koji, and other ingredients like rice and barley. Once mixed, it's fermented for at least 6 months or longer. Miso is often referred to by the ingredients used to make it or by its color. Here we'll refer to it by color.

Shiromiso (白味噌-literally white miso) has a shorter fermentation time than red miso. This results in a lighter color and flavor, with a little more sweetness than other types. Because of these aspects, I prefer using white miso for marinades and sauces.

Akamiso (赤味噌-literally red miso) is a darker miso that ranges from light brown to a dark red-brown color. Part of the color change has to do with the longer fermentation time which allows more of the Maillard reaction (natural browning) to occur. It has a much more robust flavor and I actually prefer it in my soup because of that.

You can use miso for a variety of foods, from marinating vegetables to meats and as dressing or a sauce and in soup. And if you're just starting out, the two types of miso you'll want to buy are white miso and red miso.

Tips on buying miso: When I buy miso I generally look for several things –

1. Mutenka (無添加-literally no additives) e.g. no additives like dashi. If you see dashiiri (だし入り- literally contains dashi) that means it has dashi in it. I prefer not to buy dashiiri miso so that I can use it for things aside from miso soup, e.g. the dressings in this book.
2. Yuuki (有機- literally organic)
3. Kokusan (国産-produced/grown in Japan)

Tips on using miso: like yogurt it has living bacteria (probiotics) as well as a delicate aroma that can be lost if cooked improperly (e.g. boiling in a soup). One reason miso soup comes with a lid in restaurants is to protect the aroma.

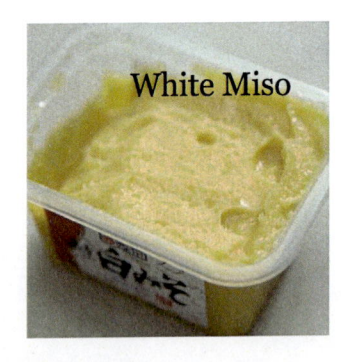

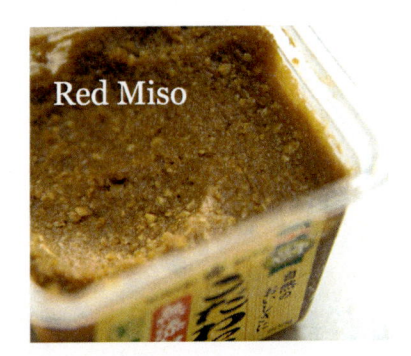

Lastly, a few words of encouragement...

I was doing part of the Shikoku Henro Trail many years ago. As I was hiking up a steep mountain trail on the way to a temple, I passed a kid and his father as they were hiking down. And I must have been huffing and puffing that made the kid cheerily say "ganbatte!" to me.

Or maybe the kid was just being a carefree kid.

Anyways, like the kid said to me, I'll say the same to you.

"Ganbatte!" (頑張って!) which loosely translated means, "keep at it!" or "don't give up!"

You got this!!

Cooking is an adventure and half the fun is making the food, smelling it, and learning!

I hope that this cookbook and my videos will help you discover new ways to cook

If you have any questions or comments, please email me at patrick@alldayieat.com, I'd love to hear from you!

PS - don't forget to get your FREE bonus materials at www.alldayieat.com/bookbonus

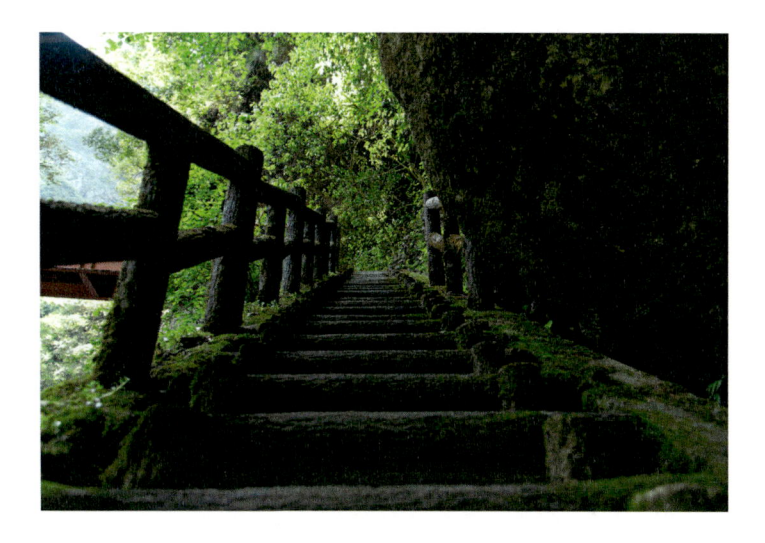

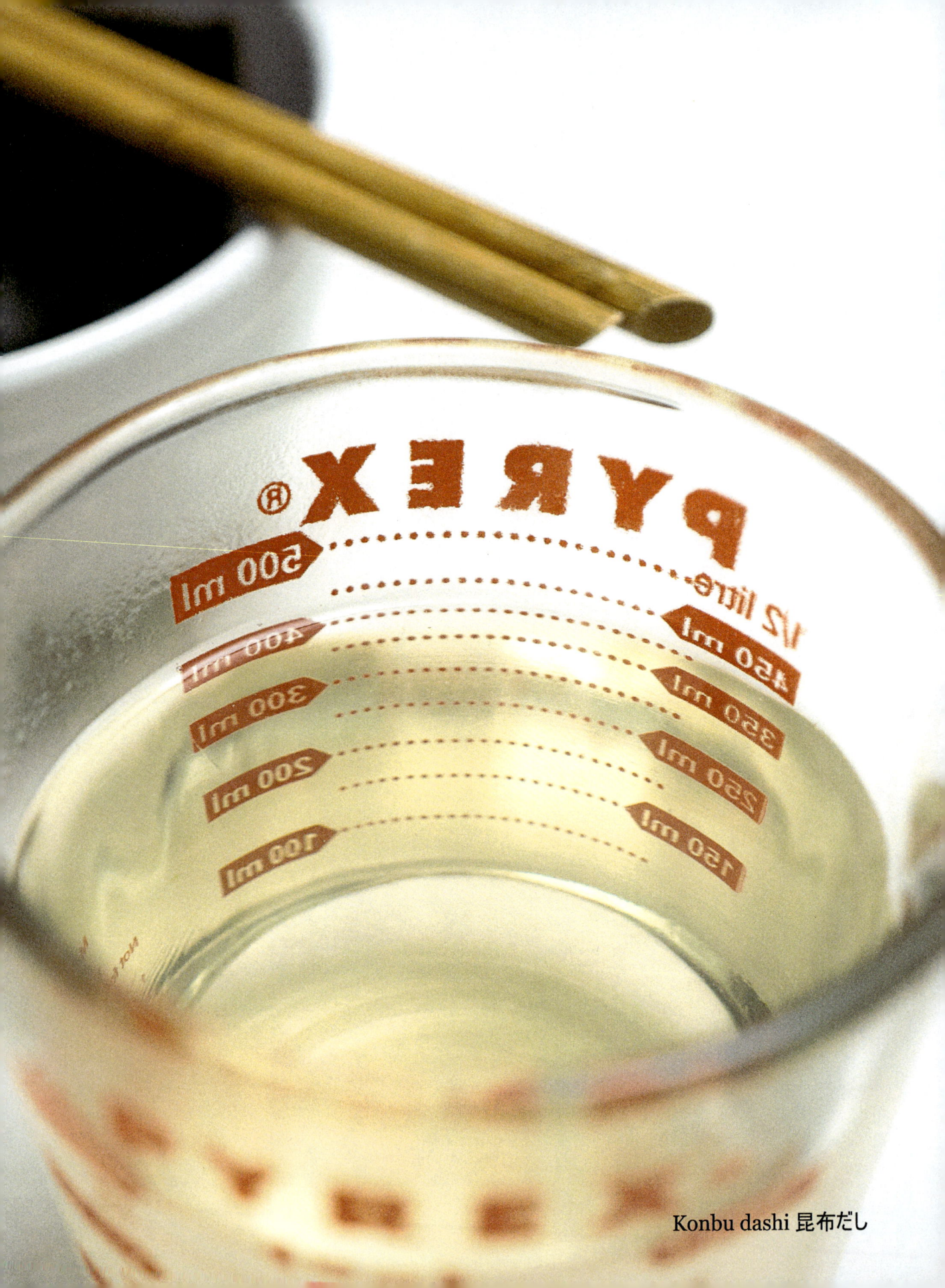

Konbu dashi 昆布だし

Konbu dashi 昆布だし

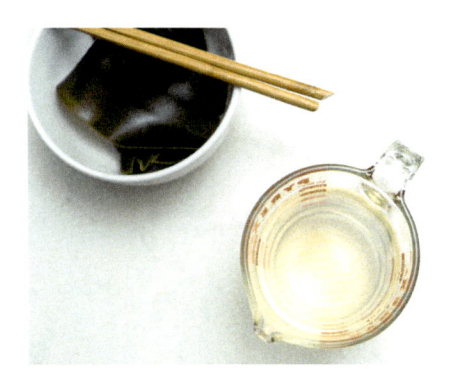

MAKES 4 CUPS

INGREDIENTS

4 x 5 in. square dried konbu (10 g)
4 cups of water

DIRECTIONS

Mizudashi (水だし cold water method)

1. Add the konbu and water to an airtight container and allow to sit in the refrigerator at least 3 hours, ideally overnight.
2. When the time has passed, strain and use immediately or store in the fridge and use or freeze within 2-3 days.
3. Save the konbu to reuse for something like tsukudani or katsuobushi dashi (see tip below).

Nidashi (煮だし simmered method)

1. Using a medium saucepan, add the konbu and water. Let it rest at least 30 minutes.
2. After time is up, heat on medium heat and bring the stock to just before a boil. You'll notice tiny bubbles forming near or around the konbu. This indicates that you'll soon need to turn the heat down and maintain that state (avoiding a boil). Keep at this level for at least 10 minutes before removing from heat.
3. Strain and use immediately or store in the fridge and use or freeze within 2-3 days.
4. Save the konbu to reuse for something like tsukudani (*recipe P. 24*).

Tips- lightly wiping dry konbu with a cloth is optional and in my experience it doesn't affect the flavor, so I don't do it. Note that the white powder you see on the konbu is the good stuff (umami). You may lose some of it if you wipe too aggressively.
- Try not to break or cut slits into your konbu as it can hasten release of bitter flavors and slime.
- For the mizudashi method, reuse the konbu a second time and add katsuobushi to make regular dashi (recipe P. 23). There's a lot of flavor left in it as the mizudashi method is passive.
- Avoid using high heat or cooking for longer than indicated. Overcooking/heating can cause bitter flavors and slime to be released into the broth.

Ichiban dashi 一番だし

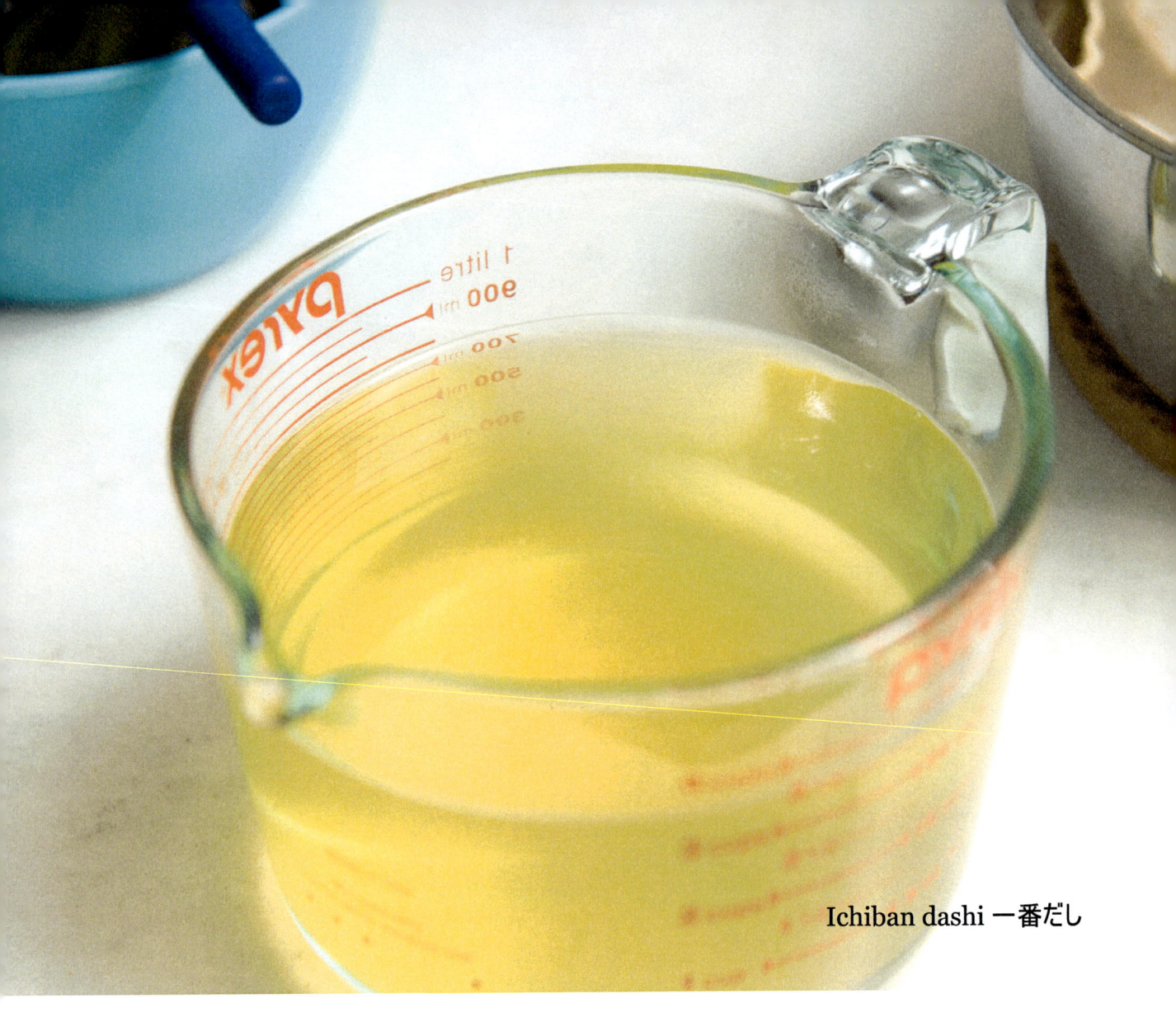

Dashi can easily be made from teabag-like dashi packets or dashi no moto (powdered dashi). But if you want a really delicious tasting dashi, you'll need to make it from scratch.

While there are many varieties and ingredients that can be used, a popular combo calls for katsuobushi flakes and konbu.

With these two ingredients, you can make ichiban dashi (dashi #1-first extraction). You can use ichiban dashi for dishes where you want to enjoy the flavor of dashi itself. For example, suimono (soup with dashi) and mentsuyu which is a noodle soup base.

For niban dashi (dashi #2-second extraction), which has less strong of a flavor, you generally use it as a base for dishes that have strong flavor components on their own. For example, nimono (simmered foods) or miso soup.

Dashi だし

MAKES 4 CUPS

INGREDIENTS

4 x 5 in. square dried konbu (10 g)
katsuobushi flakes (10 g)
4 cups of water

DIRECTIONS

For Ichiban dashi 一番だし

1. Using a medium sauce pan, soak the konbu for a minimum of 30 minutes.
2. After soaking, bring the konbu stock to barely a boil and remove from the pot. Reserve konbu for niban dashi.
3. Turn the heat up until the konbu stock begins to boil, add in the katsuobushi flakes and turn heat back down to low.
4. Simmer for 3-6 minutes.
5. Strain the katsuobushi using a paper towel lined mesh strainer, coffee filter, or nutmilk bag. *Do not squeeze the katsuobushi.*
6. You now have ichiban dashi!

For Niban dashi 二番だし

1. Return the katsuobushi from above back to the pot.
2. Add 2 cups of water and add back the same konbu used before. *Optional: add 5 grams of new katsuobushi - this is called oikatsuo (追い鰹節 - literally chasing katsuo) to add more flavor*
3. Bring the liquid to just before boiling, and turn the heat to low and allow to simmer at least 5 minutes.
4. After that time has passed, strain as before, but this time you can press against the katsuobushi.
5. Now you have niban dashi!
6. You can reuse the used katsuobushi to make furikake and you can reuse the konbu to make tsukudani, so don't throw either away!

Tips - It's important tht you avoid boiling the ichiban or niban dashi or you risk making the dashi cloudy and extracting the bitter/unwanted flavors and slime from the konbu. It's also said that some of the aromas may also be lost if the dashi is boiled.
- Both used konbu and katsuobushi can be reused after the second extraction, so try not to throw away if you like to make use of all of your ingredients.
- Try to use the dashi within 2-3 days as the flavor will soon deteriorate, if you know you won't use it, consider freezing airtight in a freezer-safe glass jar.

Sansho tsukudani 山椒佃煮

Sansho is a slightly spicy and earthy pepper. It helps to add depth and contrast to dishes that have sweet/salty flavors like unagi kabayaki (grilled eel). And by adding the pepper to soy sauce simmered konbu, you'll end up with a delicious condiment for topping tofu or white rice while ensuring your used konbu does not go to waste!

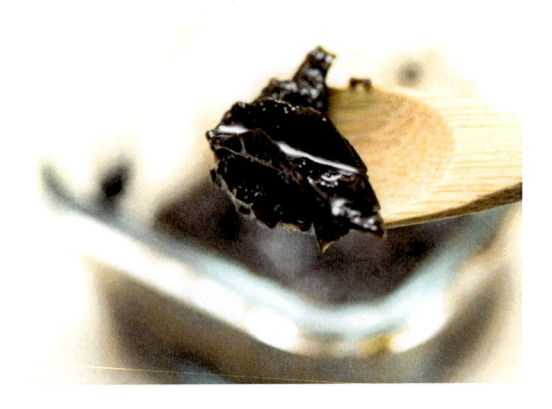

Makes 1/2 cup

Ingredients

4-6 squares of used konbu (80 g)
1 cup water
2 Tbsp rice vinegar
2-3 tsp sansho pepper
¼ cup soy sauce
1 Tbsp sugar
2 Tbsp mirin
1 Tbsp sake

Directions

1. Cut konbu into 1 in. or ½ in. squares and set aside while you measure other ingredients.
2. Combine the konbu, water, and vinegar in a small pot and heat on medium heat. Once the mixture begins to boil reduce heat to a simmer. Cover partially and cook for 15 minutes.
3. After 15 minutes, add in the rest of the ingredients and cook partially covered until liquid is reduced, 30 - 45+ minutes. The mixture will appear thick and dark.
4. You can taste for texture / wetness and remove from heat at the desired consistency. *I enjoy mine when it's like a thick glue.*
5. Store in the refrigerator airtight and use within 2-3 weeks.

Tip- If you like big chunks in your tsukudani, cut the konbu on the larger side. Smaller squares cook down better and are easier to serve.

tofu in konbu dashi

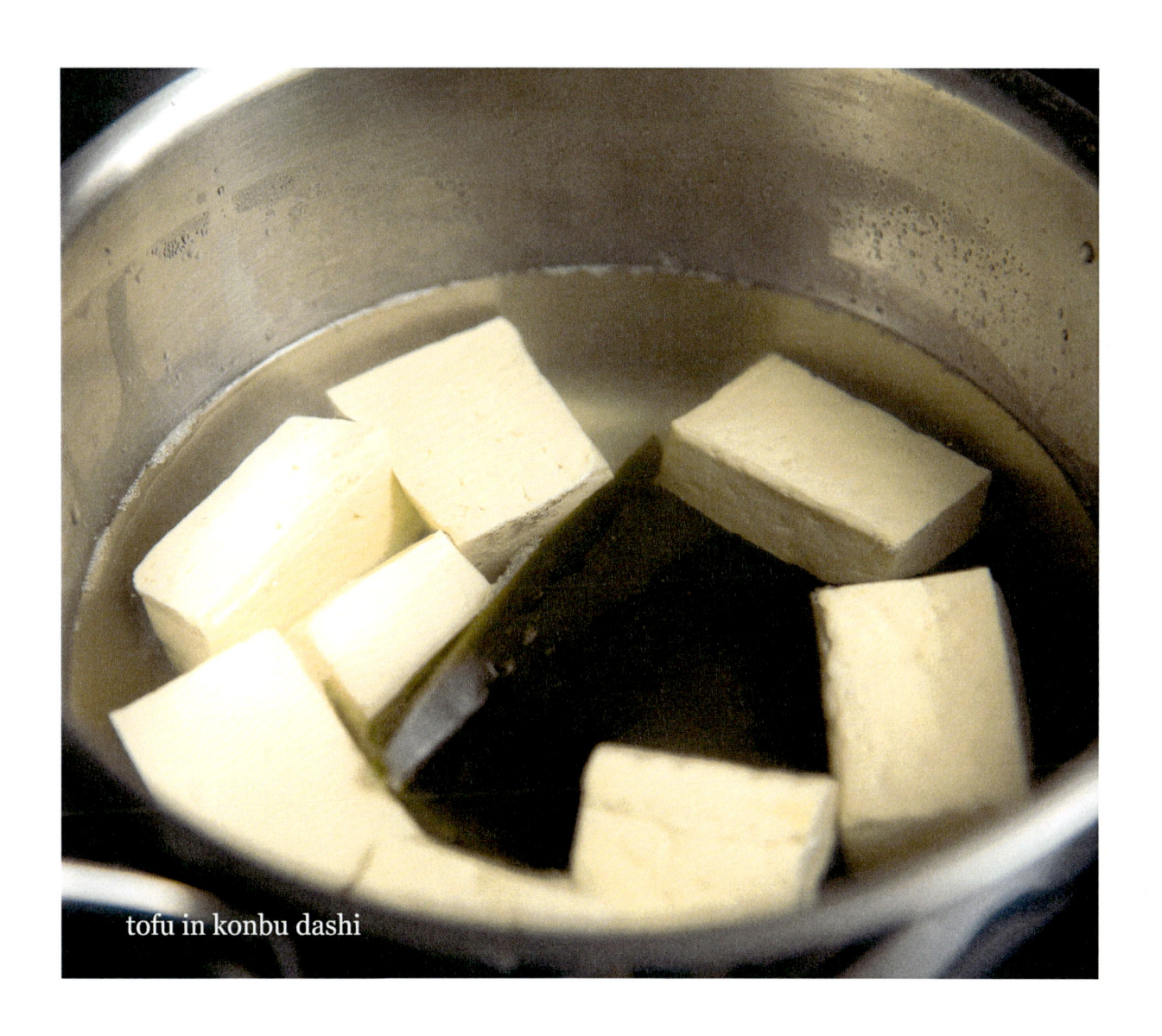

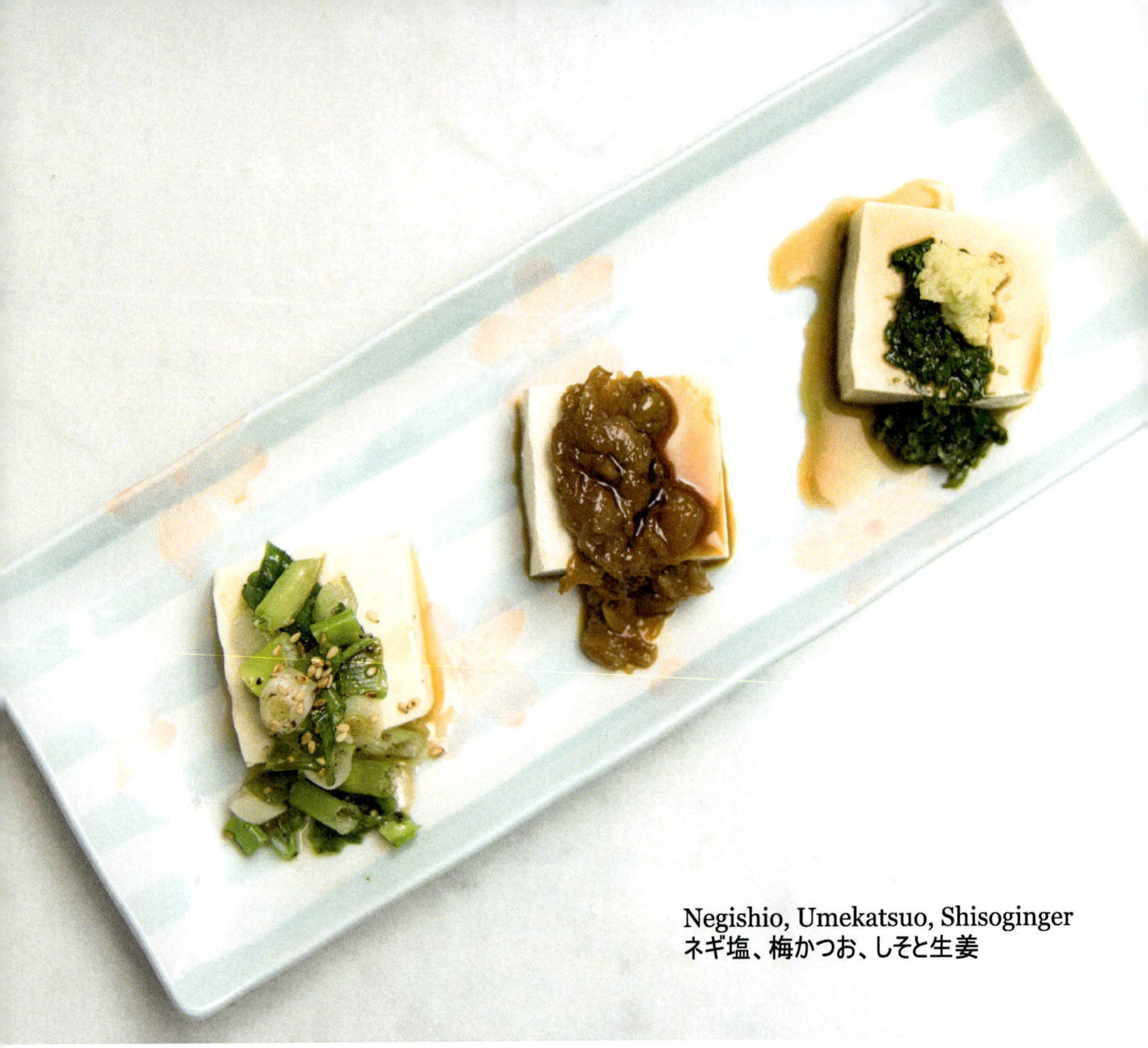

Negishio, Umekatsuo, Shisoginger
ネギ塩、梅かつお、しそと生姜

Hiyayakko 冷奴

Hiyayakko is cold tofu that not only exemplifies the delicate flavor of tofu, but also let's you enjoy a countless variety of toppings. You can even use these toppings for rice if you run out of tofu! *(Talk about emergencies!!)*

It's one of my favorite things to eat in the summer as it's not only fresh, light, and healthy, but has plenty of tofu goodness. I prefer to use soft tofu for the smooth and creamy texture.

The best part? Tofu is the vehicle for all kinds of delicious toppings. Here are 9 of my favorites.

Umejiso 梅しそ

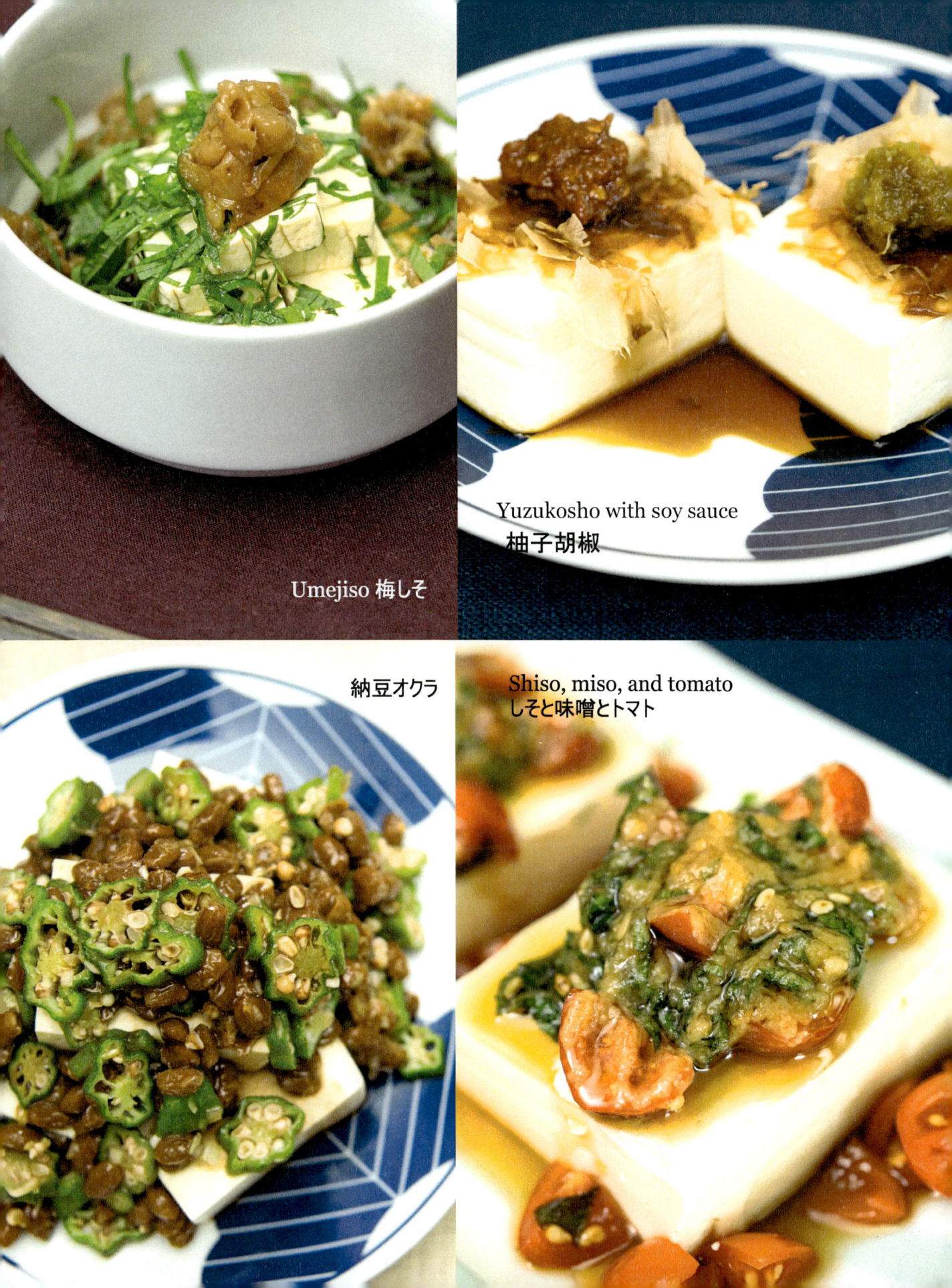

Yuzukosho with soy sauce
柚子胡椒

納豆オクラ

Shiso, miso, and tomato
しそと味噌とトマト

Negishio, umekatsuo, shisoginger hiyayakko
ネギ塩、梅かつお、しそと生姜

3 simple ways to season your tofu. The flavors here are well-balanced and help to showcase the natural flavor of the main ingredient - tofu!

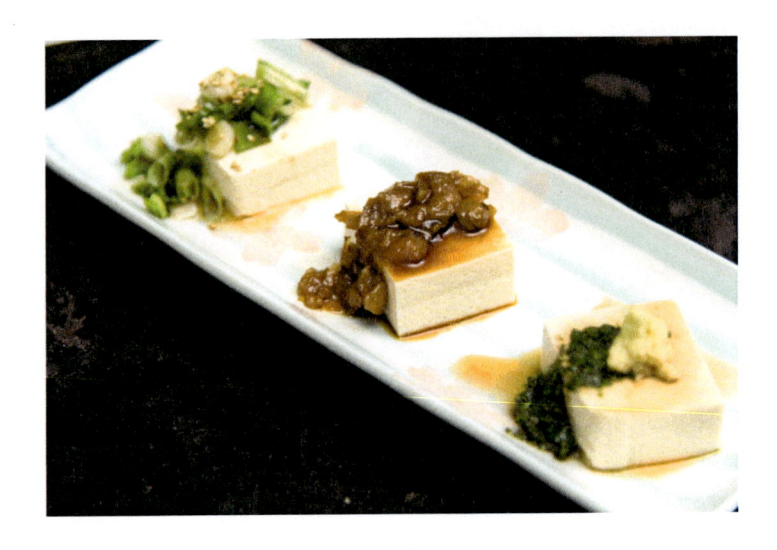

Serves 2-3

Ingredients

½ block soft tofu

Umekatsuo
2 pieces umeboshi (in shiso)
1 Tbsp katsuobushi flakes
1 tsp soy sauce

Negishio (green onion with salt)
2-3 green onions chopped
¼ tsp salt
2-3 tsp sesame oil
fresh cracked black/white pepper

Shiso ponzu with grated ginger
2 leaves shiso, chopped into thin strips
2 tsp ponzu (*recipe P. 88*)
1-2 tsp grated ginger

Directions

1. Cut tofu into squares or rectangles and plate.
2. For each of the toppings, combine in a small bowl and set aside.
3. When ready to plate, top each tofu block with toppings and serve!

Tip - wait to add your toppings to the cold tofu until just before serving. Due to the higher salt content of the sauces used, the water will get drawn out of the tofu and dilute your seasoning, especially if you forgot or didn't completely remove excess water!

Yuzukosho and sansho tsukudani hiyayakko
柚子胡椒と山椒佃煮冷奴

Two very bold ways to dress your cold tofu with soy sauce. Use yuzukosho (citrus pepper paste) or tsukudani (soy marinated kelp) and soy sauce for a simple tofu appetizer that is packed with flavor.

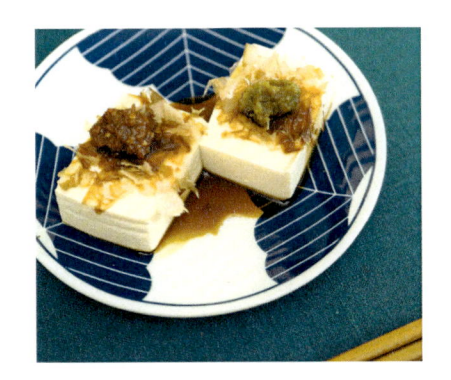

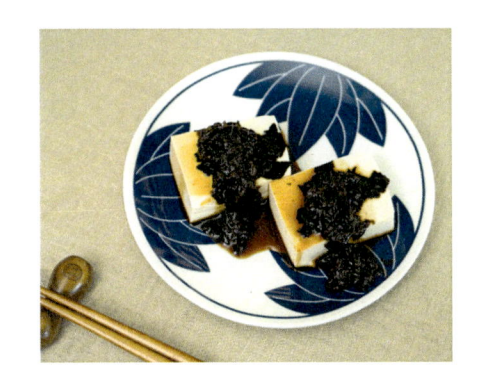

Serves 3-4

Ingredients

½ block soft tofu

For the yuzukosho
2-3 Tbsp katsuobushi flakes
2-3 tsp soy sauce
1-2 tsp red or green yuzukosho, to taste

For the sansho tsukudani
1-1½ Tbsp sansho tsukudani *recipe P. 24*
2-3 tsp soy sauce

Directions

1. Cut tofu into 2 x 3 in. rectangles and plate.
2. Top with either topping and then soy sauce to taste.

Tip - consider mixing the soy sauce with each topping, rather than drizzling over for a more balanced flavor

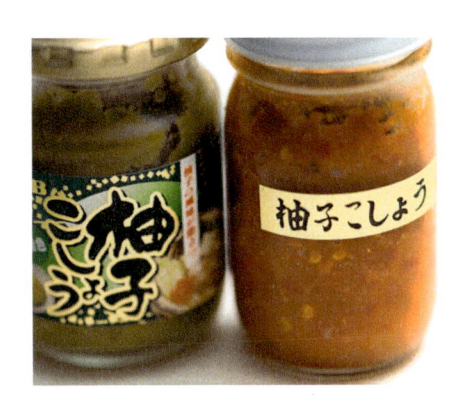

Umejiso hiyayakko
梅干しとしそ冷奴

Umeboshi (pickled plum) is often pickled with red shiso leaves. Serving umeboshi with a little green shiso and ponzu will get all the aromatics you can handle with just the right amount of tart and sour.

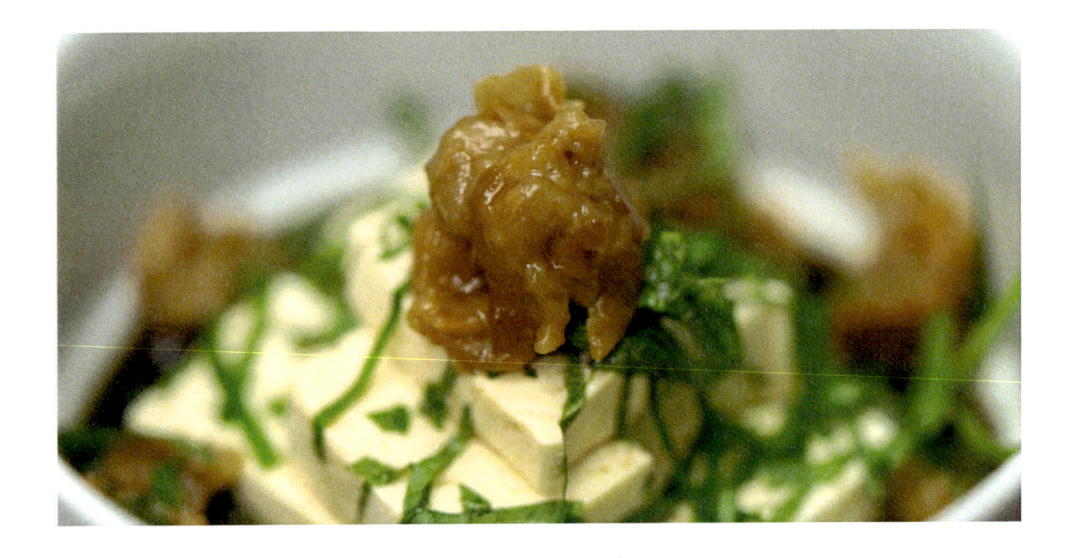

Serves 2-3

Ingredients

½ block soft tofu
3 pieces umeboshi (2-3 Tbsp)
6 leaves shiso, cut into thin strips
3 Tbsp rice vinegar
1 Tbsp soy sauce
2-3 tsp sesame oil
1 tsp sugar or ½ tsp honey

Directions

1. Cut tofu into bite size pieces and stack in a shallow bowl.
2. Separate meat from umeboshi seed and set aside.
3. Combine all remaining ingredients and half of shiso in a small bowl.
4. Pour dressing over the tofu, top with umeboshi meat, shiso and serve.

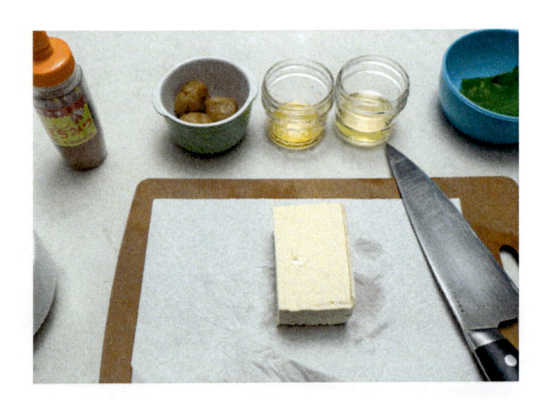

Shiso, miso, and tomato hiyayakko
しそと味噌とトマト冷奴

Shiso is one of the most fragrant and flavorful herbs used in Japanese cuisine. It works wonders on tofu. All you need are a few savory flavors to make a delicious cold tofu starter!

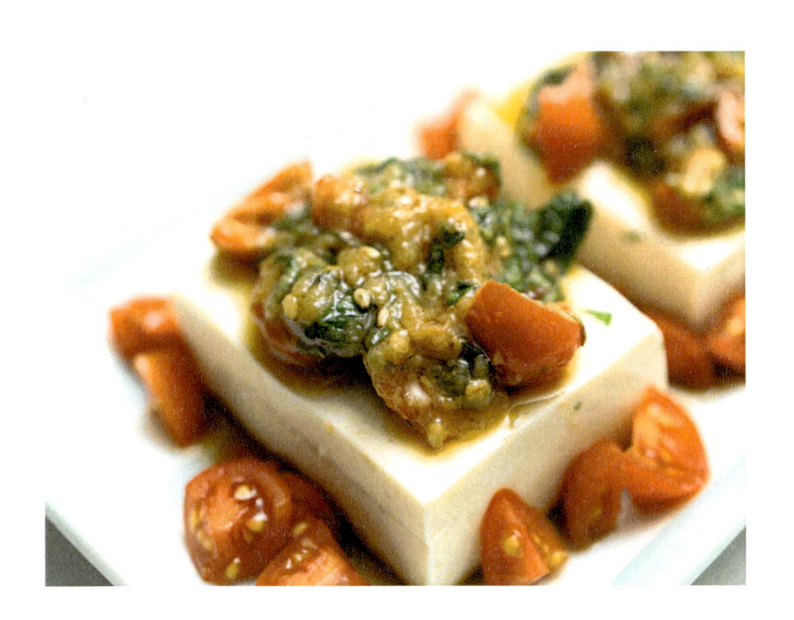

SERVES 2-3

INGREDIENTS

½ block soft tofu
10-12 cherry tomatoes, quartered
6 leaves shiso, thinly sliced
1 Tbsp white miso paste
1 Tbsp sesame oil
1 tsp mirin
1 tsp toasted sesame seeds
½ tsp honey

DIRECTIONS

1. Cut tofu into bite size pieces and put onto a serving plate.
2. Roll up shiso leaves into a small cylinder and slice thinly into small strips.
3. Combine all the remaining ingredients together, including shiso leaves, and a few tomatoes.
4. Top tofu and garnish with additional tomatoes.

Tip - Miso has varying levels of salt depending on the type and the amount used during production. Adjust for sweetness using honey or sugar with a few drops of honey or soy sauce to your liking.

Natto okra hiyayakko
納豆オクラ冷奴

Fermented soy beans with a little onion, soy sauce and blanched okra is a sticky and earthy way to top cold tofu.

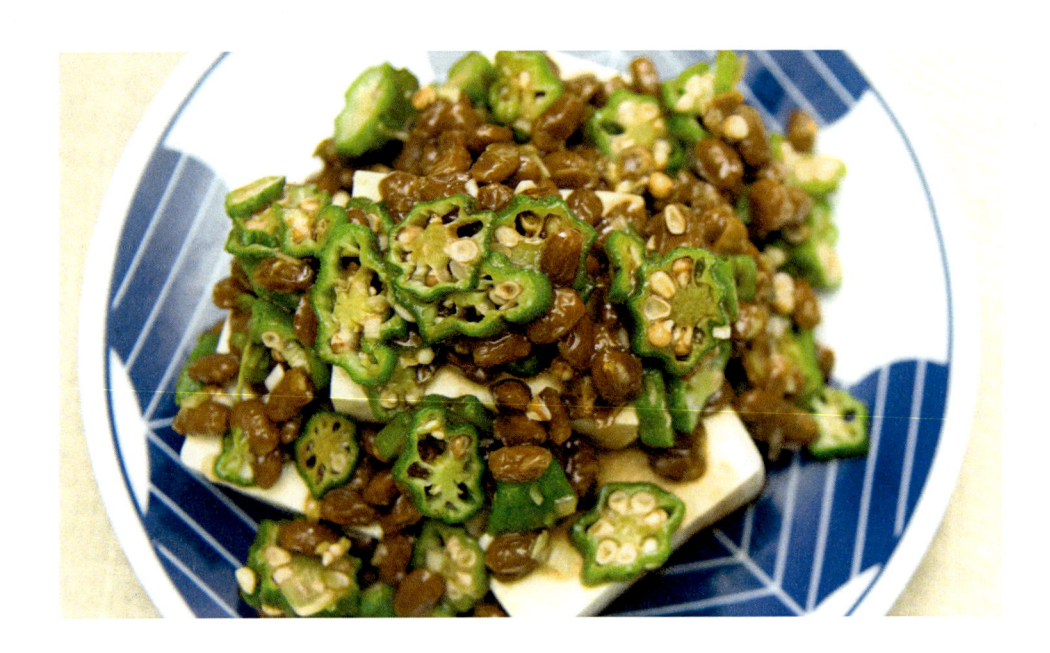

Serves 2-3

Ingredients

½ block soft tofu
1 cup okra (5-7 pieces)
3 packs natto with sauce packets or
2 tsp soy sauce
1-2 tsp katsuobushi flakes
1 Tbsp green onions, white part only, finely chopped

Directions

1. Add 1 tsp salt to a small medium sauce pan with 4 cups of water.
2. Once the water is boiling blanch okra for 1 min 30 seconds to 2 minutes max.
3. Immediately drain and shock in a cold ice water bath. *This stops cooking and helps preserve the color.*
4. Meanwhile, cut tofu into medium sized blocks and plate.
5. Once okra has chilled, thinly slice and combine with the natto, onion, and natto sauce/soy sauce.
6. Transfer the seasoned natto mixture on top of tofu and serve.

Tip- if you don't have or run out of tofu, use this to top white rice or udon noodles!

Negishiokoji hiyayakko
ねぎ塩麴冷奴

Negishio is a classic way to enjoy hiyayakko. We're making a few modest upgrades using shiokoji, sesame oil, garlic, and freshly cracked pepper.

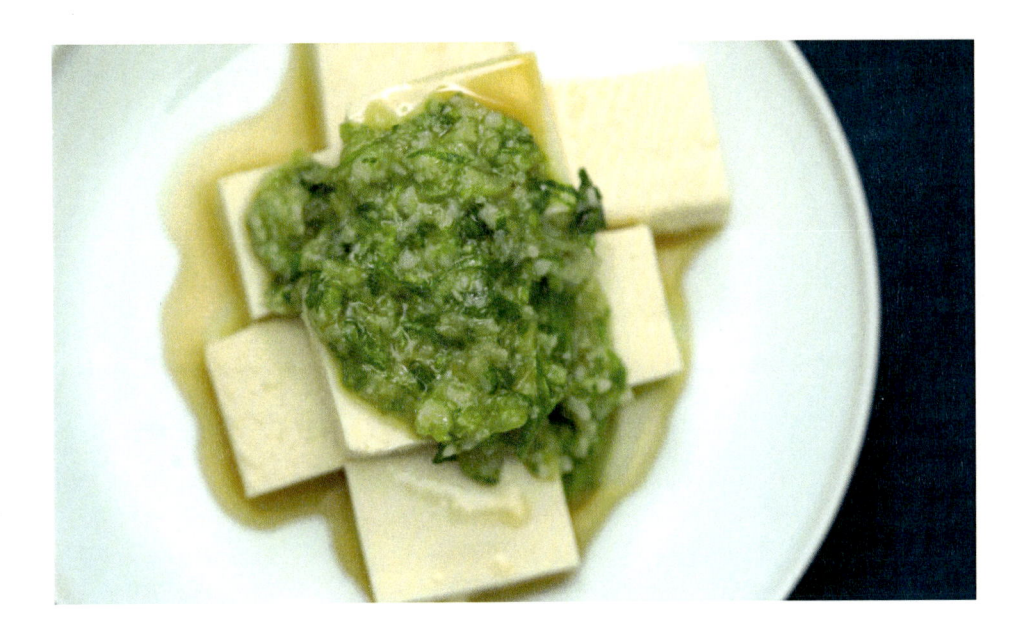

Serves 2-3

Ingredients

½ block soft tofu
1 Tbsp shiokoji
½ Tbsp sesame oil
1 clove garlic, crushed
dash of salt
1-2 stalks green onion, finely chopped
black pepper, freshly cracked
1 tsp toasted sesame seeds (optional)

Directions

1. Cut tofu into 6 large blocks and plate.
2. Prepare a small bowl and mix the topping ingredients together.
3. Spread the topping generously over the tofu and top with pepper and sesame seeds.

Tip- the negishiokojidare (negishiokoji sauce) can also be used to sauté meat such as pork, chicken, or steak. Even vegetables too!

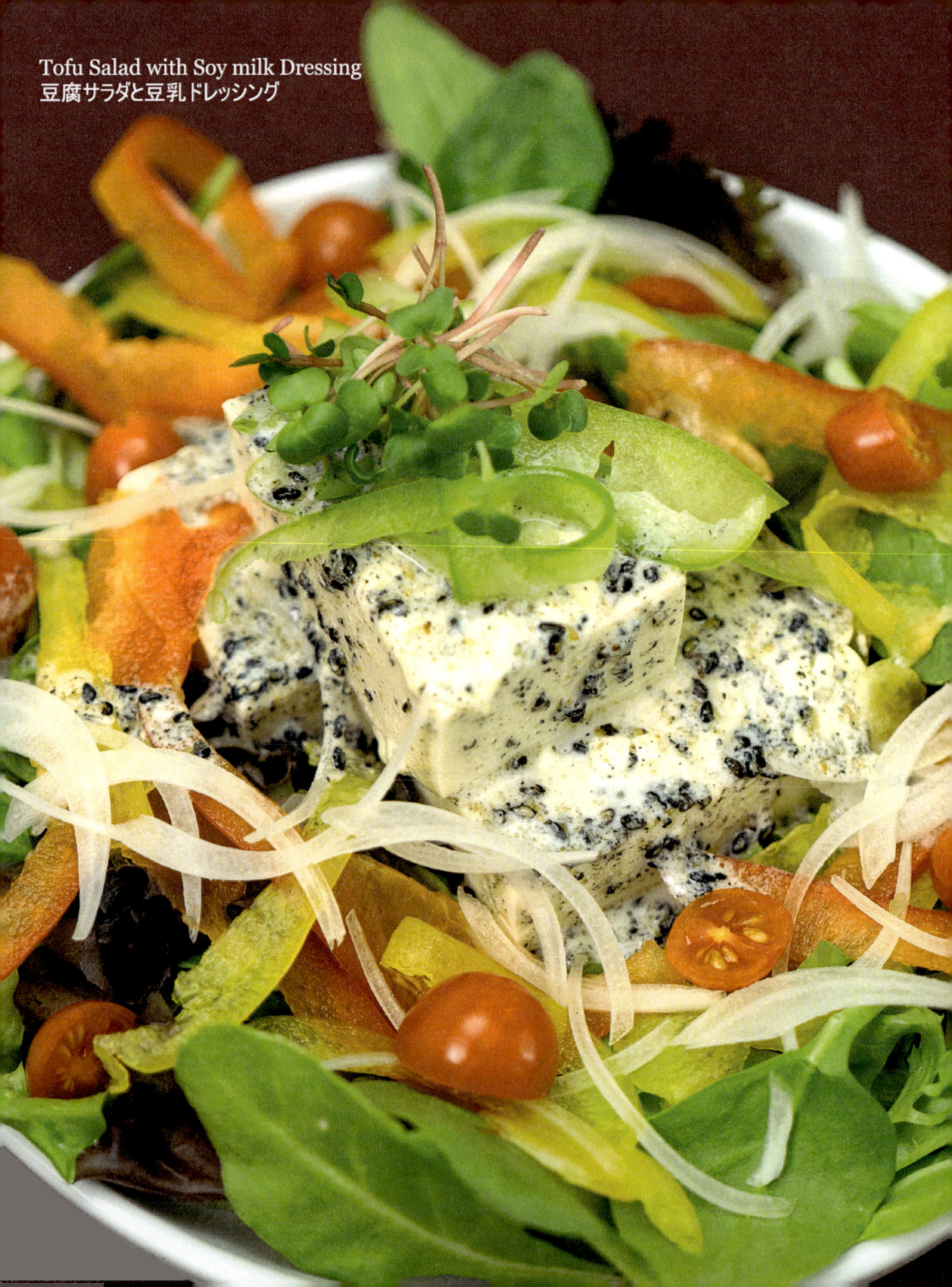

Tofu Salad with Soy milk Dressing
豆腐サラダと豆乳ドレッシング

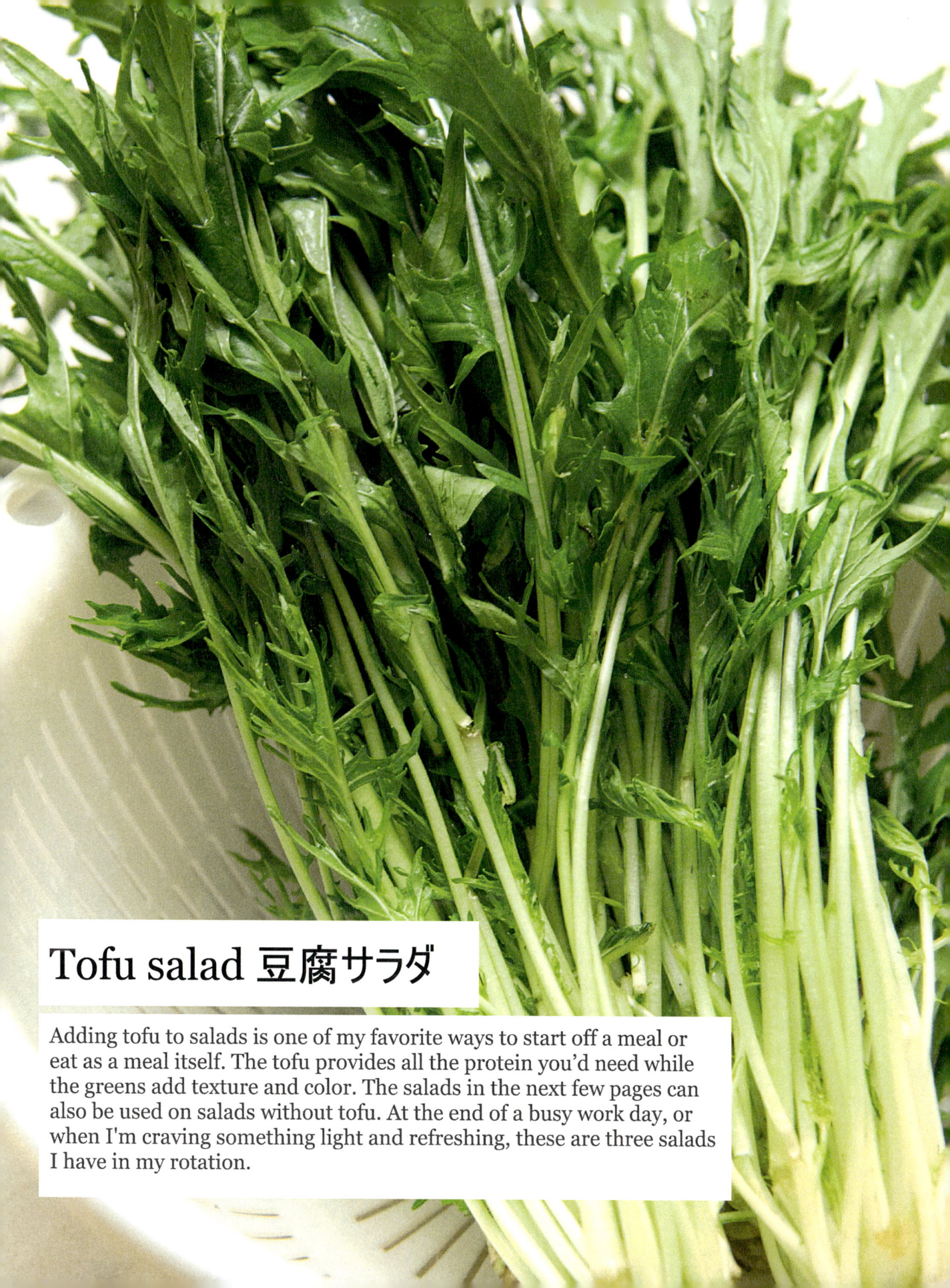

Tofu salad 豆腐サラダ

Adding tofu to salads is one of my favorite ways to start off a meal or eat as a meal itself. The tofu provides all the protein you'd need while the greens add texture and color. The salads in the next few pages can also be used on salads without tofu. At the end of a busy work day, or when I'm craving something light and refreshing, these are three salads I have in my rotation.

Tofu salad with sesame vinaigrette
豆腐サラダと胡麻ドレッシング

This is a very light dressing that can work well on greens alone, I add slices of tofu to make it a light meal.

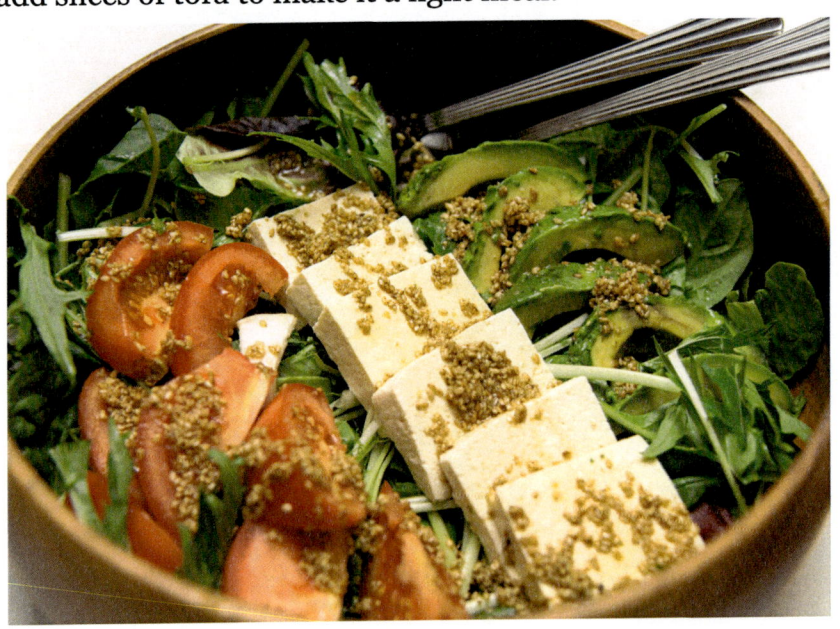

SERVES 3-4

INGREDIENTS

½ block soft tofu
½ avocado, sliced
2-3 tomatoes, quartered
5 oz baby greens
½ bunch mizuna

For the dressing
¼ cup white sesame seeds, toasted
4 Tbsp rice vinegar
2 Tbsp extra-virgin olive oil
2 tsp sesame oil
1 Tbsp soy sauce
2 tsp sugar or 2 tsp honey
¼ tsp salt
1-2 Tbsp water to thin, optional

DIRECTIONS

1. Combine all ingredients under dressing and mix thoroughly.
2. Cut tofu block into bite site pieces.
3. Using a large bowl, layer greens, followed by tofu blocks, tomatoes, avocado, and dressing.
4. Toss before serving.

Notes - For an extra nutty/sesame flavor add another tablespoon of ground sesame seeds

- I also enjoy this with the tomato, avocado, and tofu without any greens.

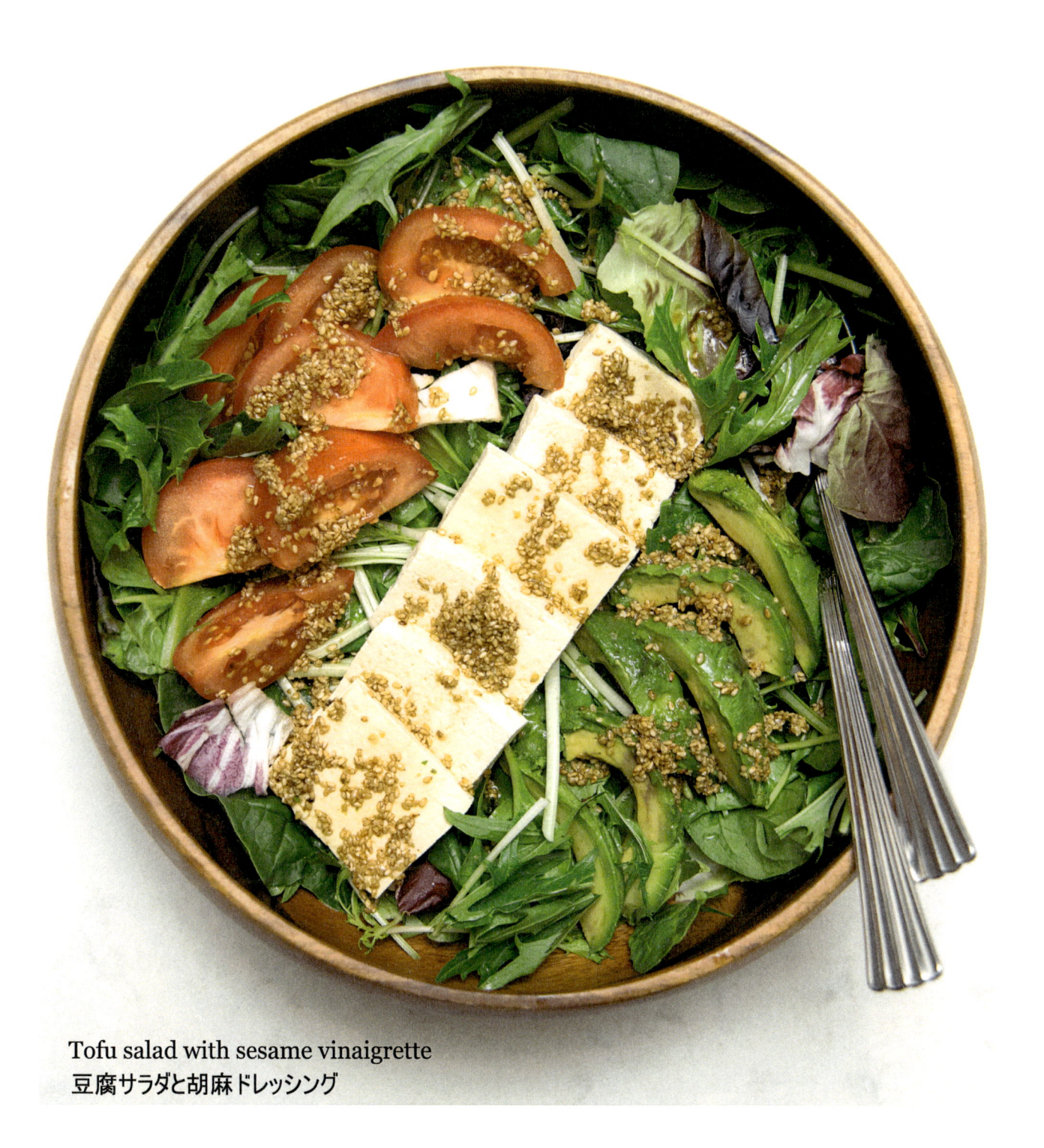

Tofu salad with sesame vinaigrette
豆腐サラダと胡麻ドレッシング

Tofu salad with gomadare
豆腐サラダとごまだれ

This gomadare is a rich dressing that's creamy, nutty, and savory. Miso paste and ground sesame seeds are a magical combo that work wonders on this and many other baby green based salads!

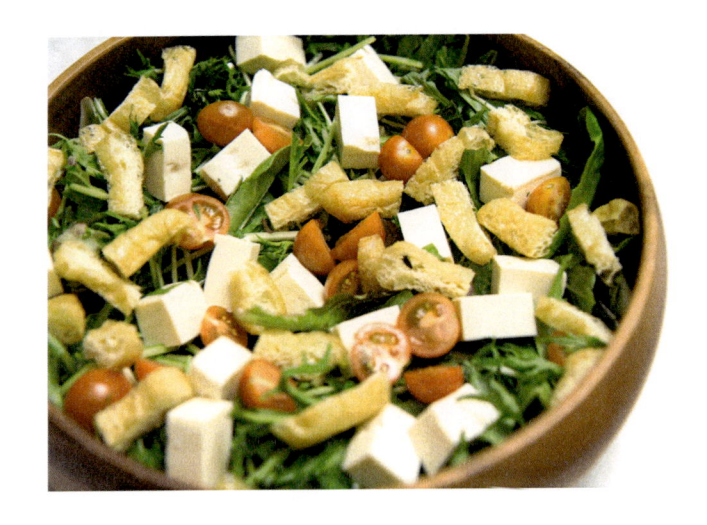

SERVES 3-4

INGREDIENTS

½ block soft tofu
5 oz baby greens
½ bunch mizuna
10-12 cherry tomatoes or 2-3 whole tomatoes quartered
2 pieces aburaage (fried tofu skin)

For the dressing
¼ cup white sesame seeds, toasted and ground
4 tsp miso paste
4 tsp mayonnaise
4 tsp soy sauce
2 tsp sesame oil
1 tsp sugar or ½ tsp honey

Optional 1-2 tsp sesame seeds

DIRECTIONS

1. Combine all ingredients under dressing and mix thoroughly.
2. Cut tofu block into bite size pieces.
3. Using a large bowl, layer greens, followed by tofu blocks, tomatoes, aburaage, and dressing.
4. Toss before serving.

Tips - if you enjoy crunchy textures with your salad, toast the aburaage in your toaster or on a cast iron pan for 1-2 minutes until crispy. Alternatively, broil your tofu pieces in the oven for 2-3 minutes for a warmer version of this salad!

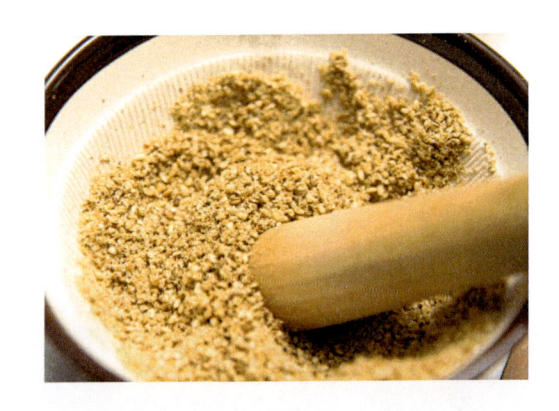

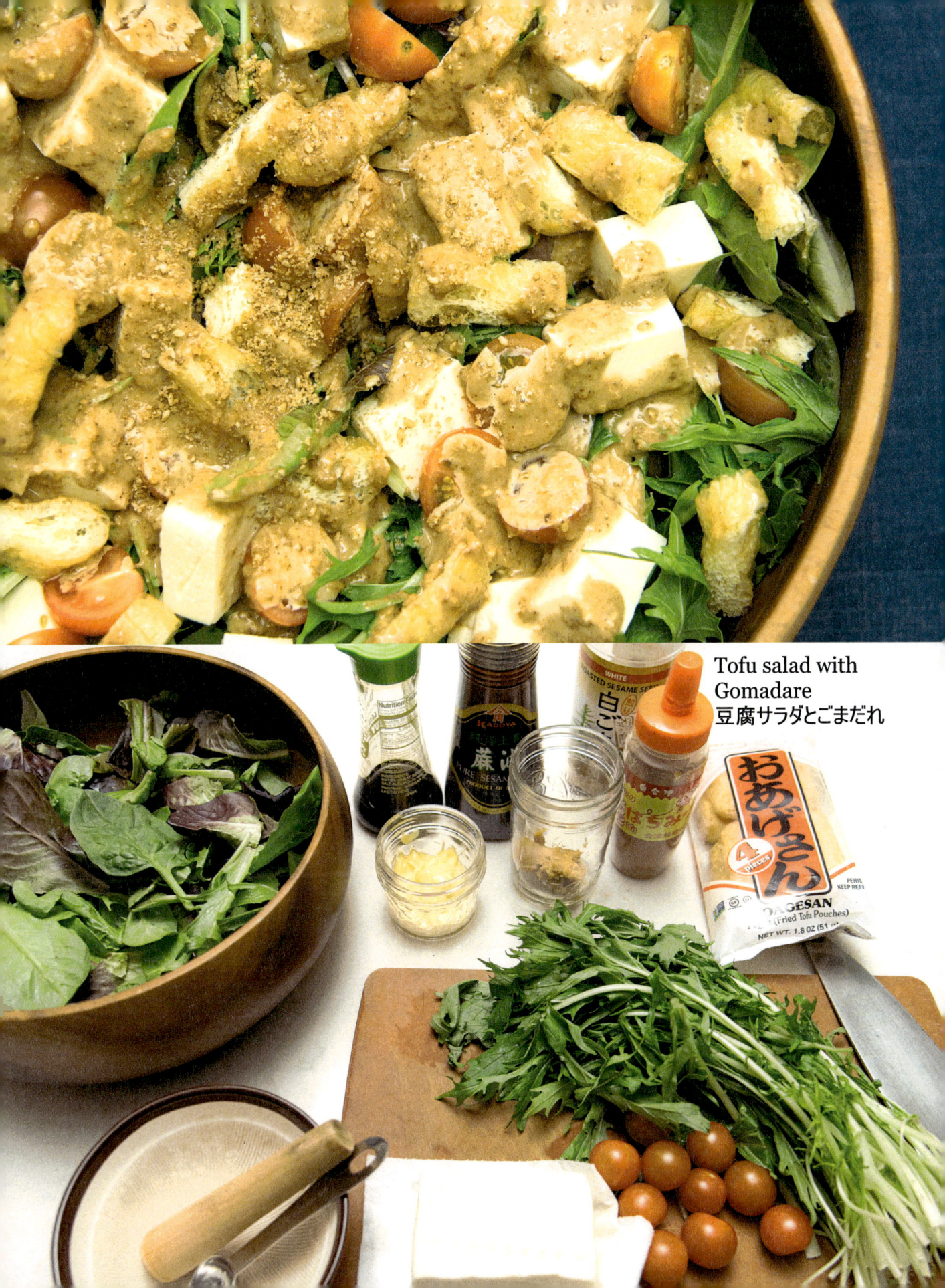

Tofu salad with Gomadare
豆腐サラダとごまだれ

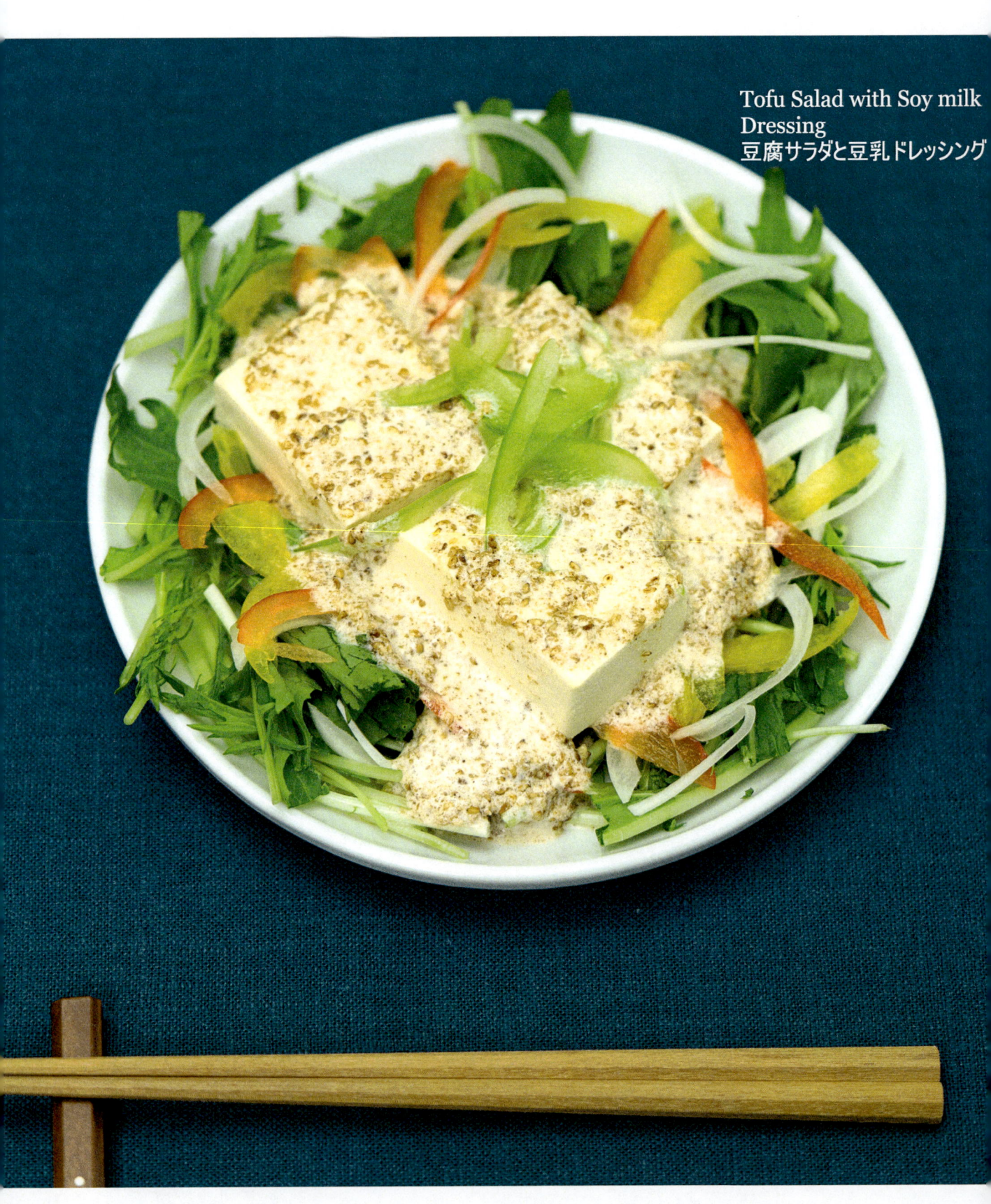

Tofu Salad with Soy milk Dressing
豆腐サラダと豆乳ドレッシング

Tofu salad with soy milk dressing
豆腐サラダと豆乳ドレッシング

This is an extremely light and nutty dressing that's full of flavor. You can use it on greens alone, tofu alone, or a combo. Alternate white and black sesame seeds for a little variation, or combine them both!

Serves 2-3

Ingredients

1 block soft tofu
2 cups konbu dashi *recipe P. 21*
¼ cup each of red, yellow and green bell pepper, thinly sliced
¼ cup white onion, thinly sliced
2-3 handfuls of mizuna
2-3 handfuls of baby greens or arugula

For the dressing
2-3 Tbsp sesame seeds, toasted and ground
2-3 Tbsp lemon juice
1 tsp honey
1 tsp salt
2 Tbsp Kewpie mayonnaise
2 Tbsp sesame oil
½ cup soy milk (unsweetened unflavored)

Directions

For the dressing
1. Mix all ingredients into a large bowl or canning jar and mix thoroughly.
2. If needed, add a few drops of honey, dash of salt or 1-2 tsps lemon juice to taste.

For the salad
1. Cut the tofu into bite size cubes or flat squares.
2. Using a small pot with konbu dashi cook tofu for at least 15 minutes, drain, and set aside. *This step is optional but adds another layer of flavor and umami.*
3. Use a mandolin or knife to thinly slice bell peppers and onion.
4. Use a medium plate and spread a layer of baby greens and chopped mizuna and top with tofu blocks.
5. Drizzle soymilk dressing and garnish with bell peppers.

Tips - mix things up and use black sesame seeds for a different color!
- For a richer dressing, increase the mayonnaise by a Tbsp and decrease sesame oil by an equal amount.

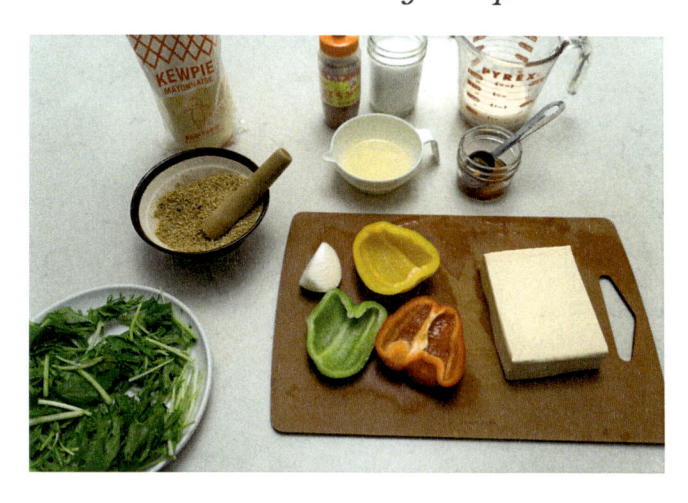

Asparagus shiraae
アスパラ白和え

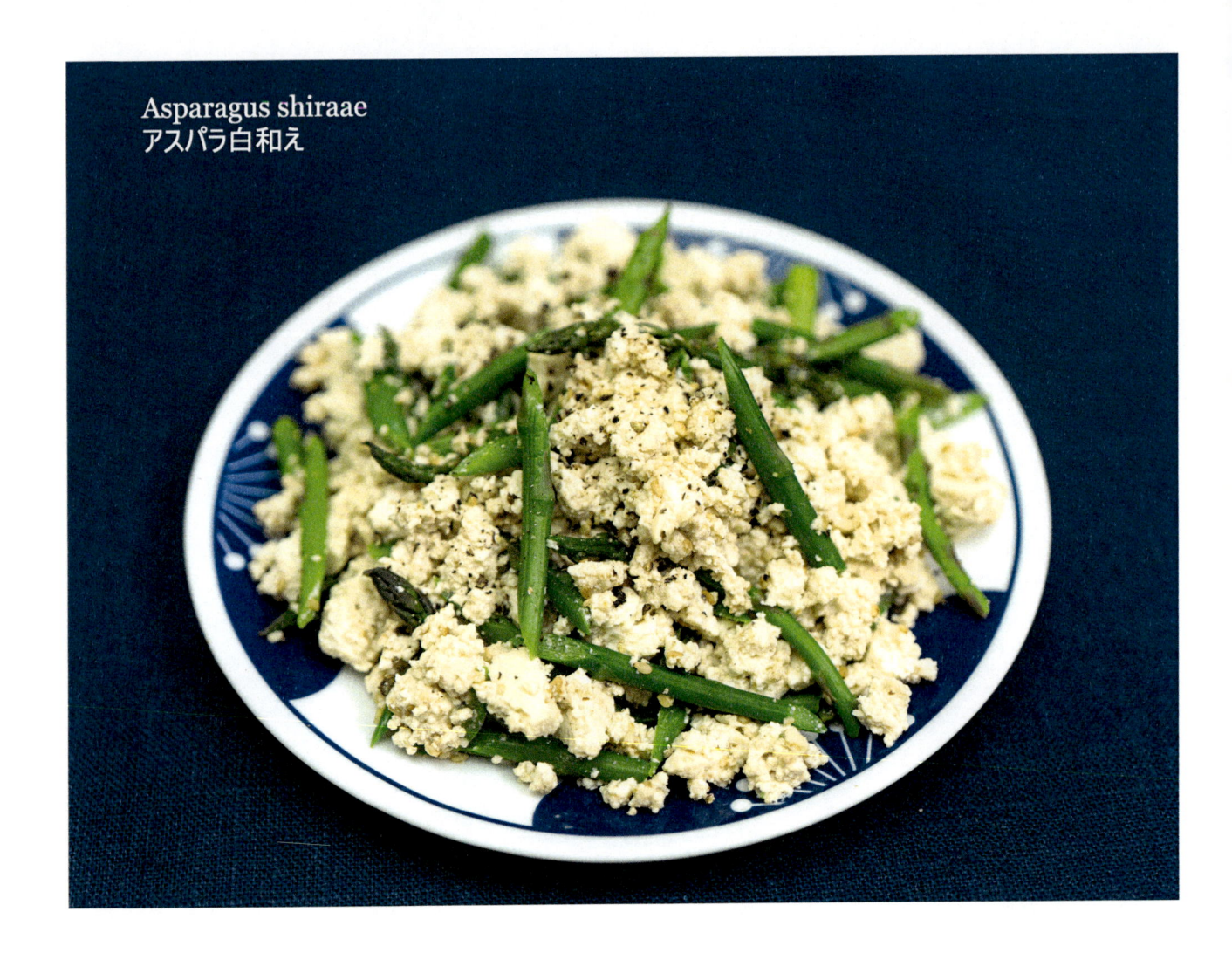

Shiraae 白和え

At its most basic, shiraae is made with sesame seeds, soy sauce, and tofu. This forms a rich and creamy base that is nutty, savory, and serves as the base flavor for the vegetables you have in season.

There are many variations and things you can add to your shiraae base, but two of the more common call for dashi stock and miso paste.

I used to prefer shiraae cold, but after being impatient and not allowing the vegetables to cool, eating it slightly warm grew on me. Perhaps, you'll like it that way also!

The next few pages illustrate some of my favorite ways to season my vegetables. The shiraae way!

toasted white sesame seeds

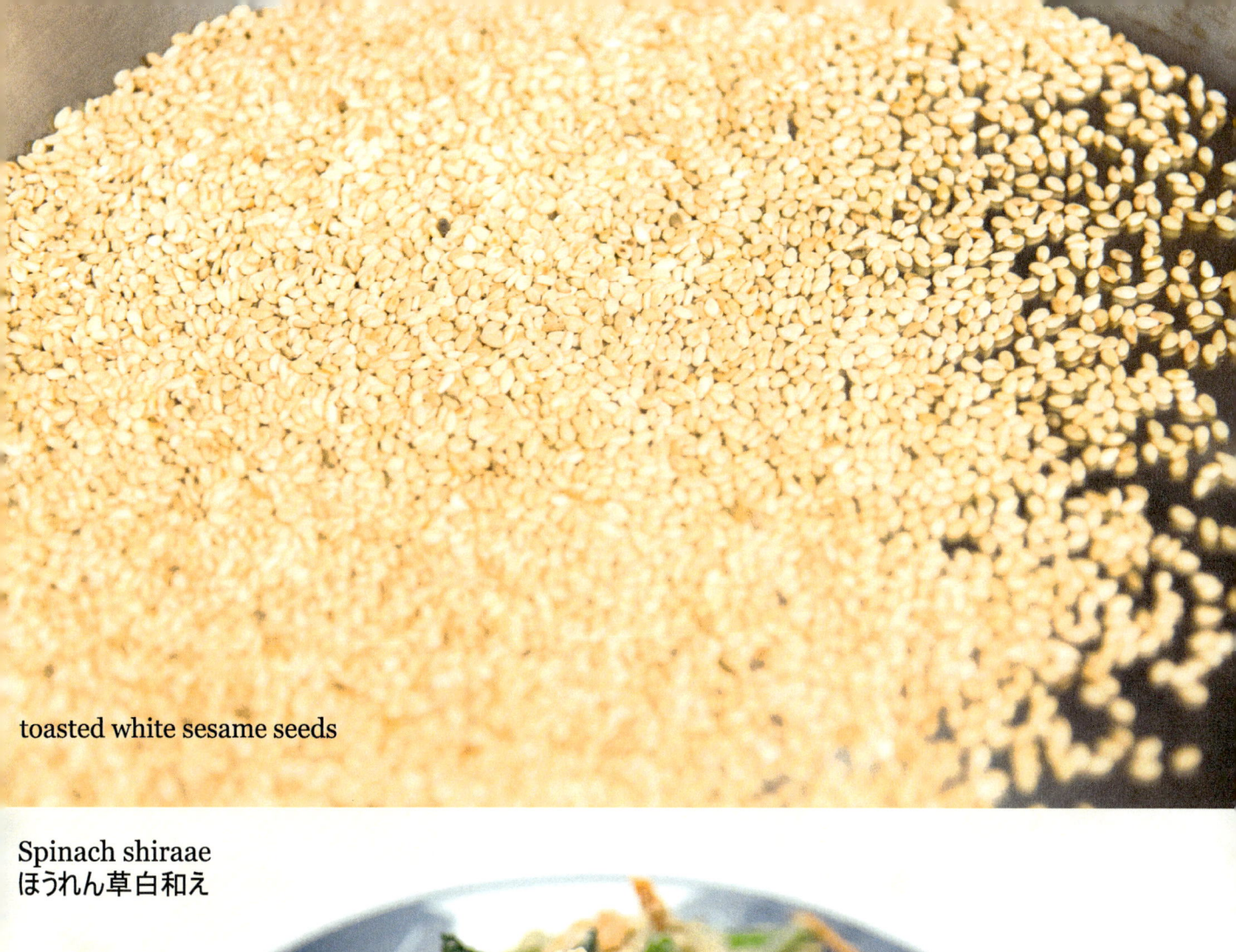

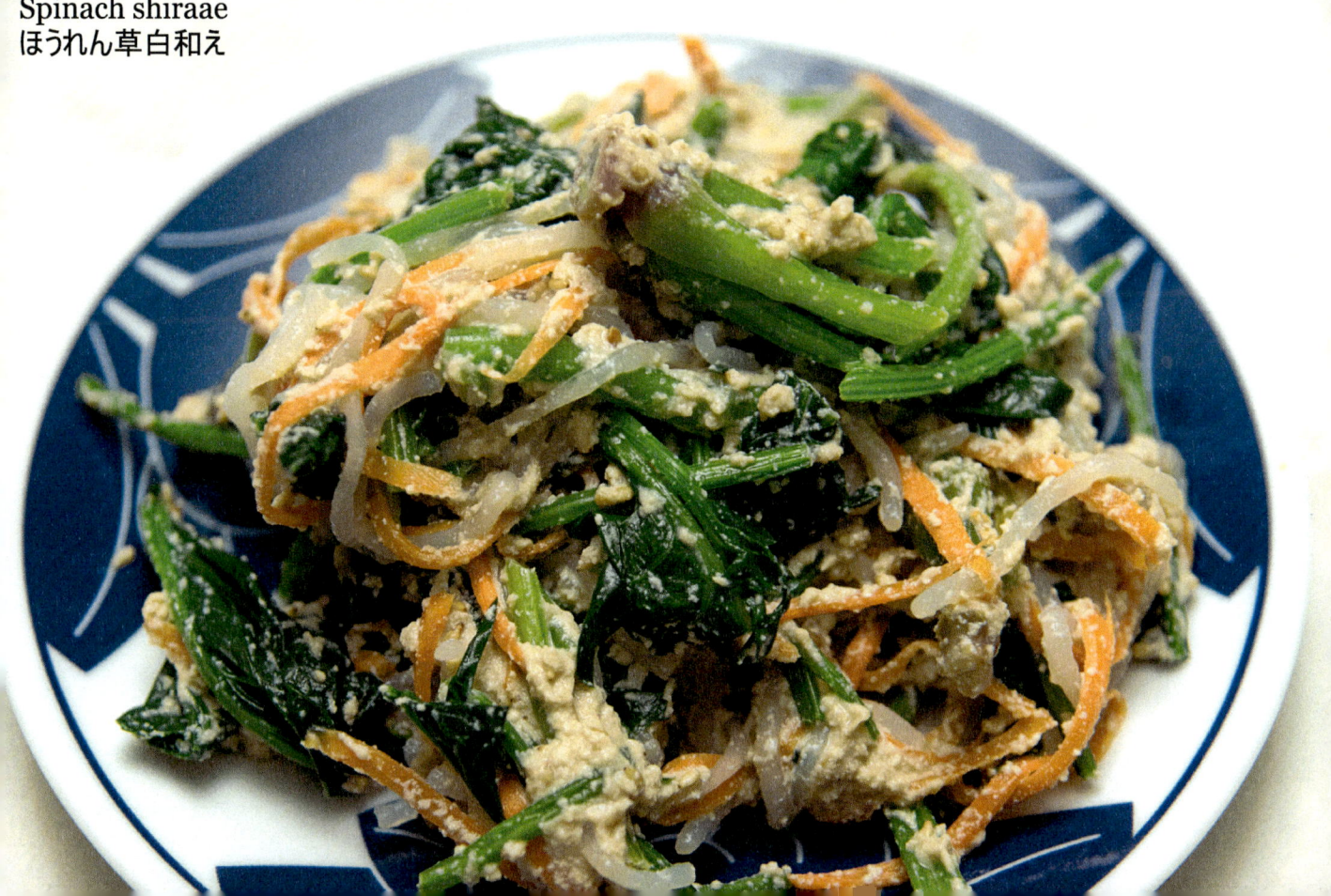

Spinach shiraae
ほうれん草白和え

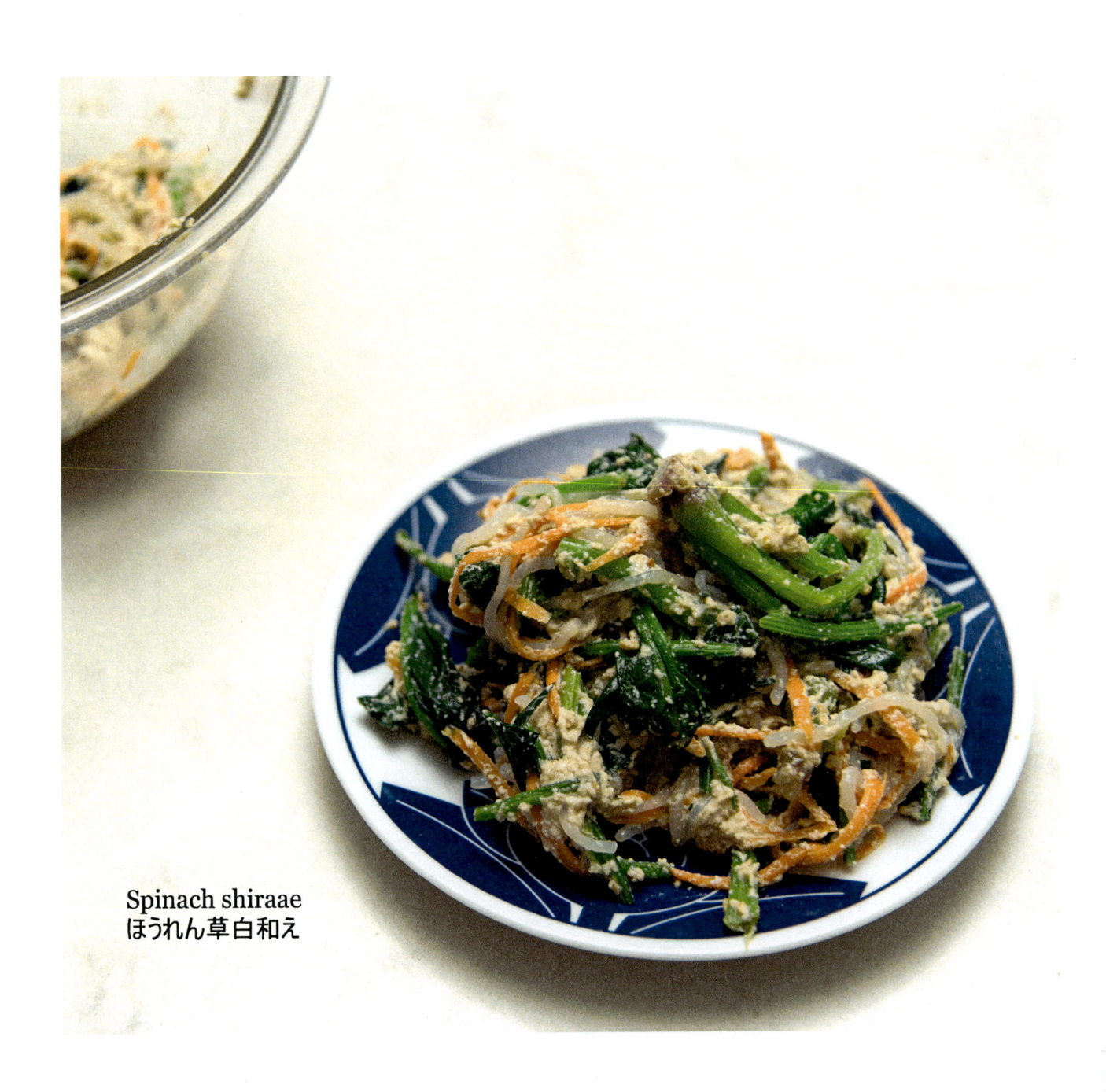

Spinach shiraae
ほうれん草白和え

Spinach shiraae ほうれん草白和え

This is an extremely light shiraae that's full of flavor and a little on the savory side, just the way I like it! Spinach, carrot, and shirataki are one of my favorite combinations. Even better, it's something you can eat year-round. Consider switching the white sesame seeds with black for a different flavor and presentation!

Serves 4

Ingredients

½ block firm tofu
1 bunch spinach
1 package white shirataki noodles (7 oz.), noodles cut in half
2-3 carrots shredded, about one heaping cup

Shiraae mixture
1½-2 tsp light soy sauce
2 Tbsp white sesame seeds, toasted
2 tsp sugar

Directions

1. Prepare a large pot of boiling water and blanch the carrots and shirataki for about a minute and 30 seconds.
2. Once cooked, scoop the carrots and shirataki noodles into a strainer and drop in an ice bath to cool.
3. Using the same water, add the spinach and blanch for a minute. Then drain and shock with cold water.
4. Once spinach has cooled, cut into 1-2 in. sections and squeeze out water. Set aside in a large mixing bowl.
5. Meanwhile, use a food processor to process tofu, sesame seeds, soy sauce, and sugar. Process until smooth or slightly chunky, if desired.
6. Squeeze excess water from carrots and shirataki noodles.
7. Combine tofu mixture with the vegetables and serve.

Tip – light soy sauce (usukuchi shoyu) helps to preserve the light off-white color of the shiraae, it has a higher salt content than regular soy sauce (shoyu), but is less likely to affect the natural color of the food it seasons.

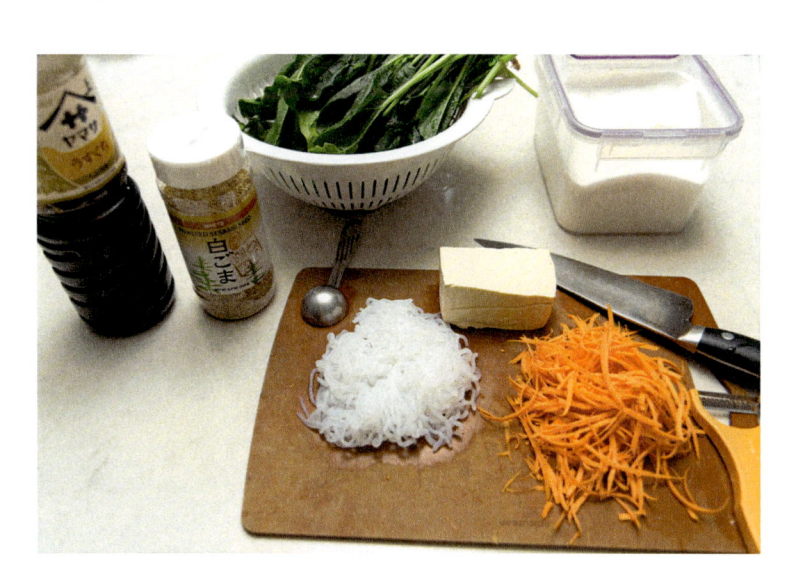

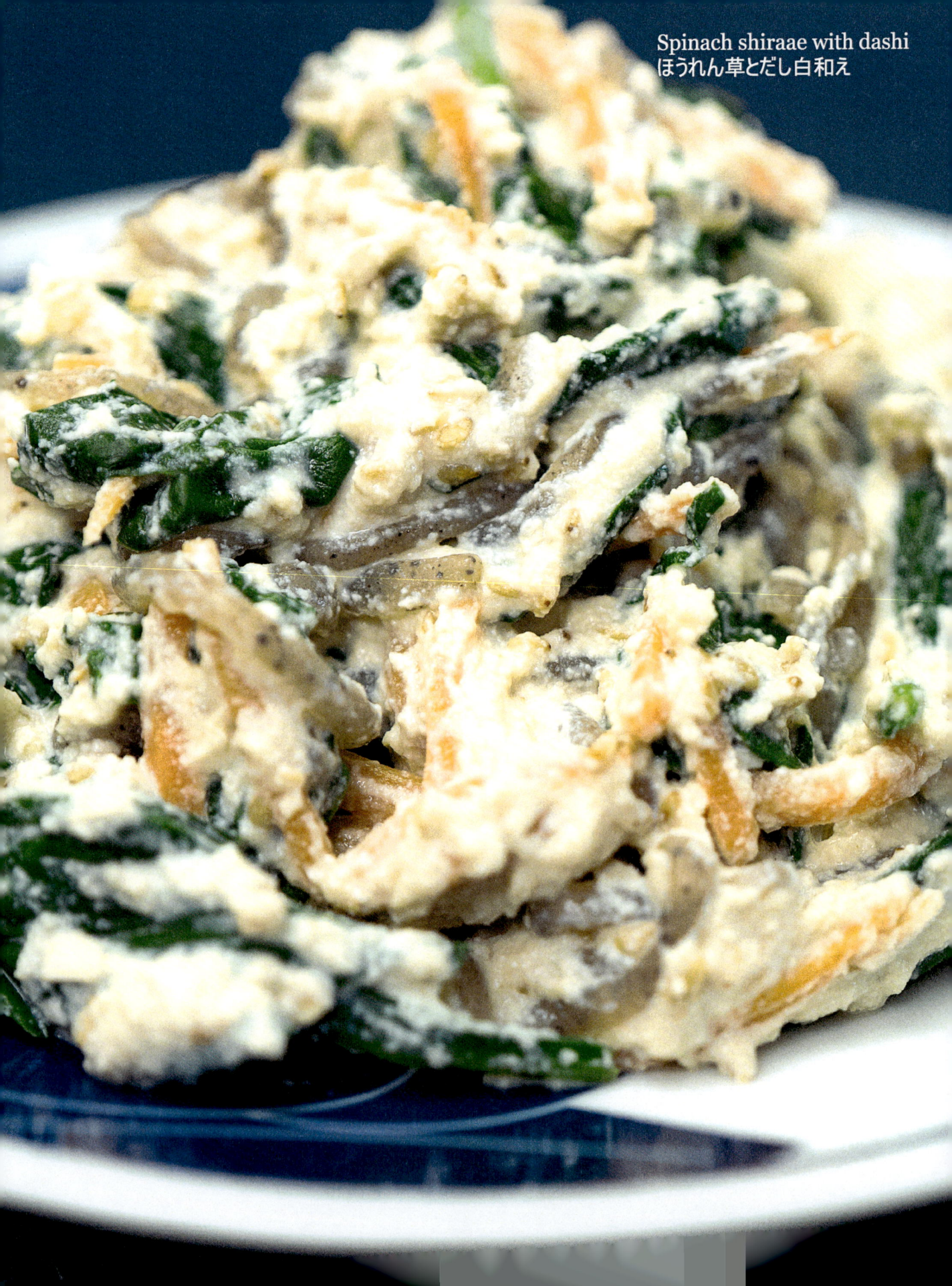

Spinach shiraae with dashi
ほうれん草とだし白和え

Spinach shiraae with dashi
ほうれん草とだし白和え

If you want a shiraae with a more complex flavor, just add dashi. This version is a little saucier with a very different flavor profile than the previous shiraae recipe. A good way to keep your shiraae fresh and new.

Serves 4

Ingredients

½ block firm tofu
1 bunch spinach
1 package shirataki noodles (7 oz.), noodles cut in half
2-3 carrots shredded, about one heaping cup

Dashi mixture
½ cup dashi, *recipe P. 23*
2 tsp soy sauce
2 tsp mirin

Shiraae mixture
2 Tbsp white sesame seeds, toasted
1 Tbsp light soy sauce (usukuchi shoyu)
2 Tbsp mirin

Directions

1. Prepare a large pot of boiling water and blanch the spinach and shirataki for a minute.
2. Drop in the ice bath and allow to cool.
3. Once spinach has cooled, squeeze out water and cut into small sections about 2 inches or ¼ of the length. Set aside in a large mixing bowl.
4. Add the carrots and shirataki to a small pot and add the dashi mixture. Cook for about 4-5 minutes and remove from heat.
5. Use a strainer and drain carrots and shirataki into another pot; allow to cool. *See note for reusing liquid.*
6. Meanwhile, use a food processor to process tofu, sesame seeds, soy sauce, and mirin. Once processed to the desired consistency, add to bowl with spinach.
7. Combine tofu spinach mixture with the vegetables and serve.

Tip - Save the dashi, soy, mirin marinade for something else like soba, udon or gomaae!

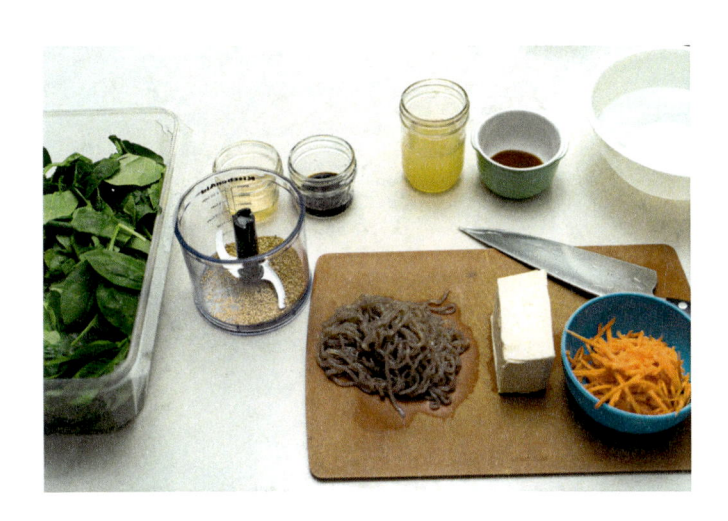

Green bean shiraae インゲン白和え

This green bean shiraae is one of the lightest and simplest you can make. If you're looking for a quick and easy way to enjoy green beans Japanese style this might be a good way to start!

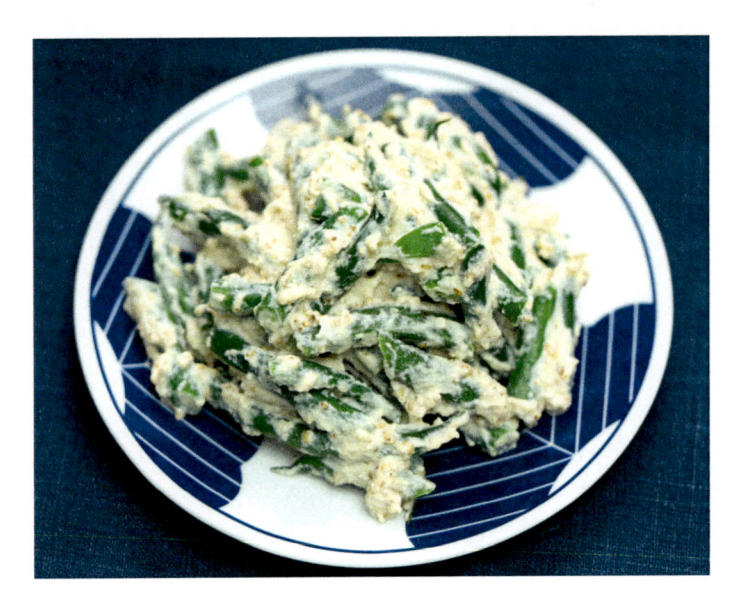

Serves 4

Ingredients

½ block soft tofu
½ lb. green beans, trimmed
3 Tbsp sesame seeds, toasted
1 Tbsp sugar
1 ½- 2 tsp light soy sauce (usukuchi shoyu)

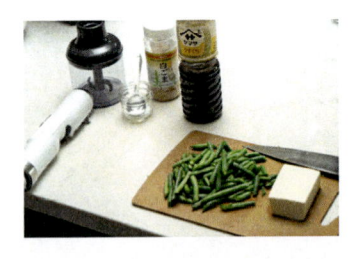

Directions

1. Cut green beans into 1-2 in. pieces.
2. Prepare a large pot of boiling salted water and blanch your green beans for 1-2 minutes until desired firmness.
3. Shock with cold running water and/or an ice bath.
4. Dry thoroughly using a paper towel or tea towel.
5. While the green beans are cooking you can start on the seasoning.
6. Add sesame seeds, sugar, and light soy sauce to a food processor and process 15-20 seconds. Then add the tofu and process another 20-30 seconds until it has a slightly rough texture. Set aside.
7. Once green beans have cooked and cooled, add to a large bowl.
8. Add the tofu mixture to the green beans and mix thoroughly.
9. Serve with additional sesame seeds. Salad can be served slightly chilled or at room temp.

Asparagus shiraae アスパラ白和え

Asparagus lends itself well to rice and pasta based dishes, so it's only natural that it works well with tofu! What makes this shiraae special is that we use white miso paste to add a few layers of flavor and umami!

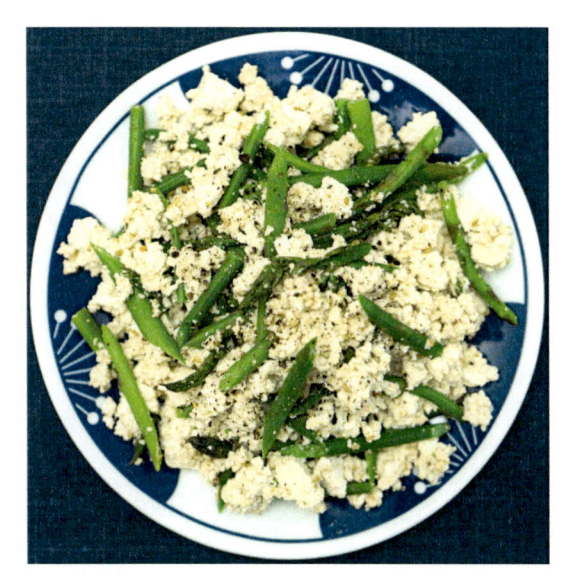

Serves 4

Ingredients

½ block firm tofu
½ bunch asparagus (4oz)
2 tsp light soy sauce (usukuchi shoyu)
1 tsp white miso paste
1-2 drops of honey or 1 tsp sugar
1 Tbsp white sesame seeds, toasted ground
black pepper, freshly cracked

Directions

1. Prepare a medium pot of lightly salted boiling water and blanch asparagus for 1 minute and 30 seconds. Immediately drain and shock in a cold ice bath.
2. Cut cooled asparagus into 1-2 in. pieces at a sharp angle.
3. In a food processor or suribachi, grind the sesame seeds.
4. Then add soy sauce, miso paste, and tofu. Grind lightly until evenly mixed or to desired consistency. *I like this with some small chunks of tofu leftover*.
5. Mix in asparagus and top with black pepper.

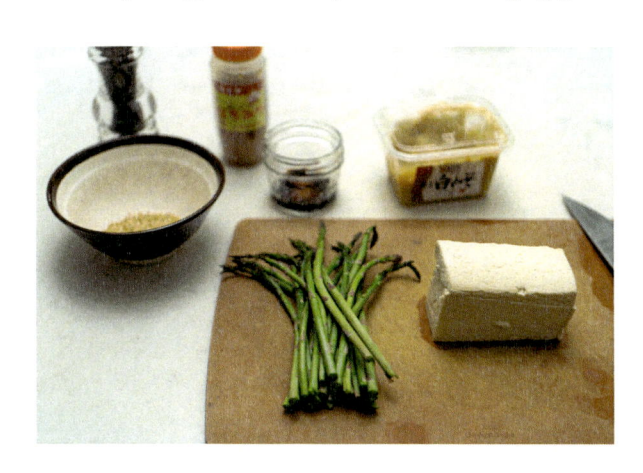

Ankakedoufudon
あんかけ豆腐丼

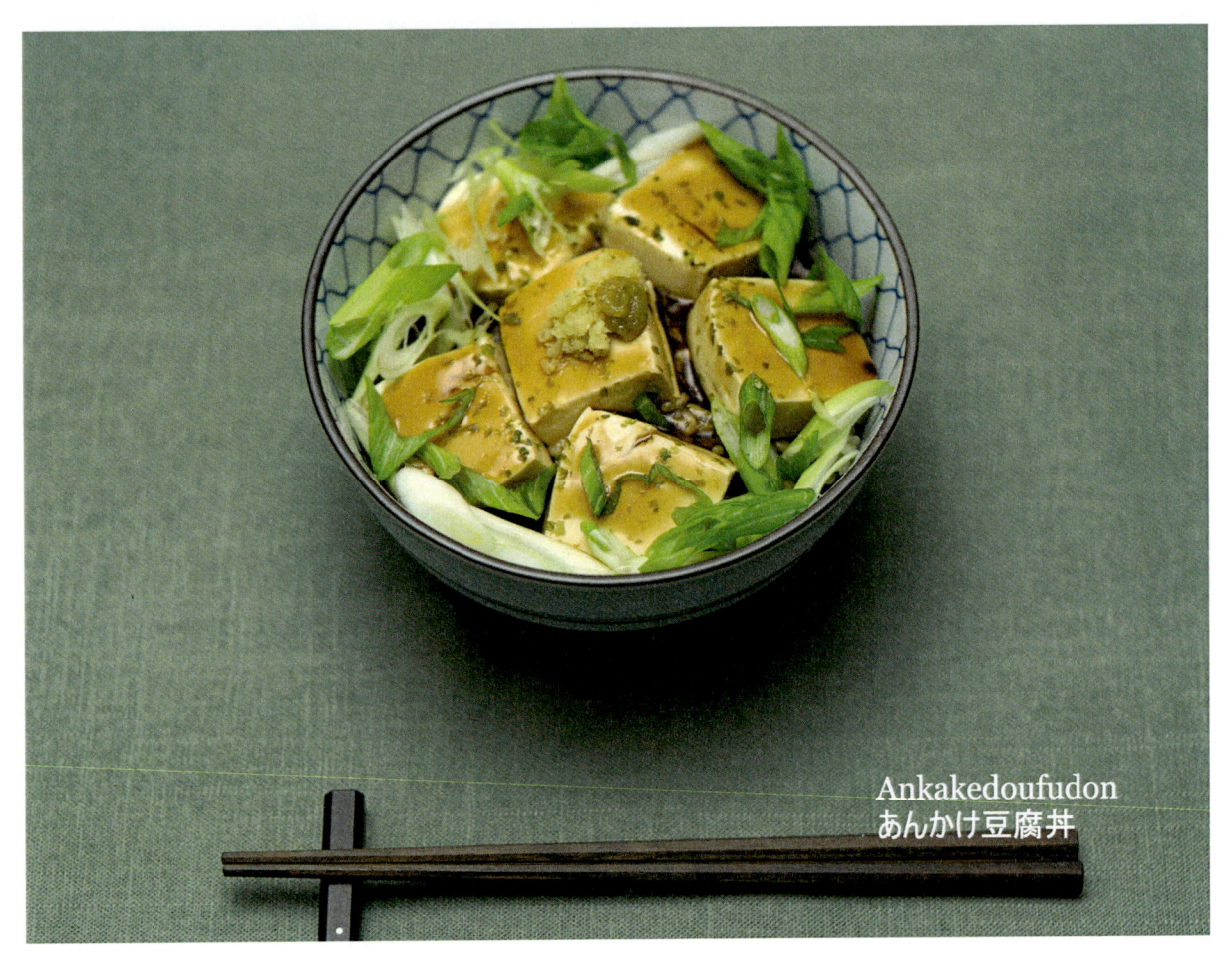

Warm tofu dishes

In this next section, we're going to cover a few of my favorite warm tofu recipes. These include misodengaku (味噌田楽), ankakedoufu (あんかけ豆腐), atsuage (厚揚げ), karaage (唐揚げ), pan-fried tofu steaks, and cubes.

The misodengaku is one of my go-to miso sauces and can be used for other vegetables like eggplant and konnyaku.

The ankakedoufu recipes can be adapted and served on top of a bowl of rice to make it a 'donburi'. Also, note that the technique of thickening a sauce with potato starch is not limited to tofu either, you can use 'an' sauce for noodles, vegetables, meats, and fish too!

Lastly, we'll finish up with a few deep-fried and pan-fried dishes. Though I don't eat deep-fried tofu often, when I do, karaage and atsuage are the top two ways I enjoy it.

If you're watching your calorie or oil intake, consider broiling the tofu. Like the dengaku recipe, the tofu steak recipes can easily be modified by broiling the uncoated tofu steaks for 2-3 minutes with a similar end result. Haven't tried it yet? Maybe now's the time!

Karaage 唐揚げ

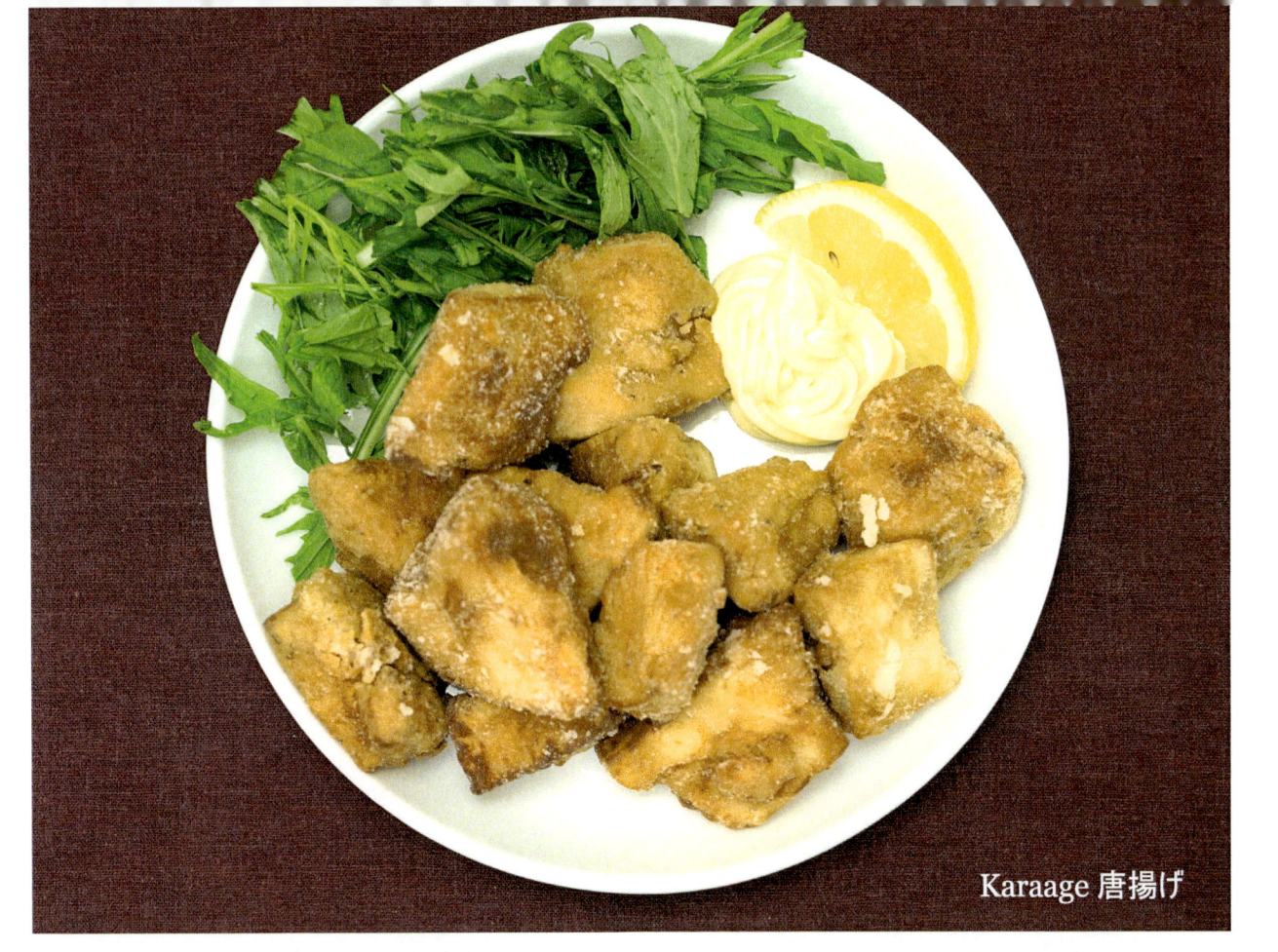

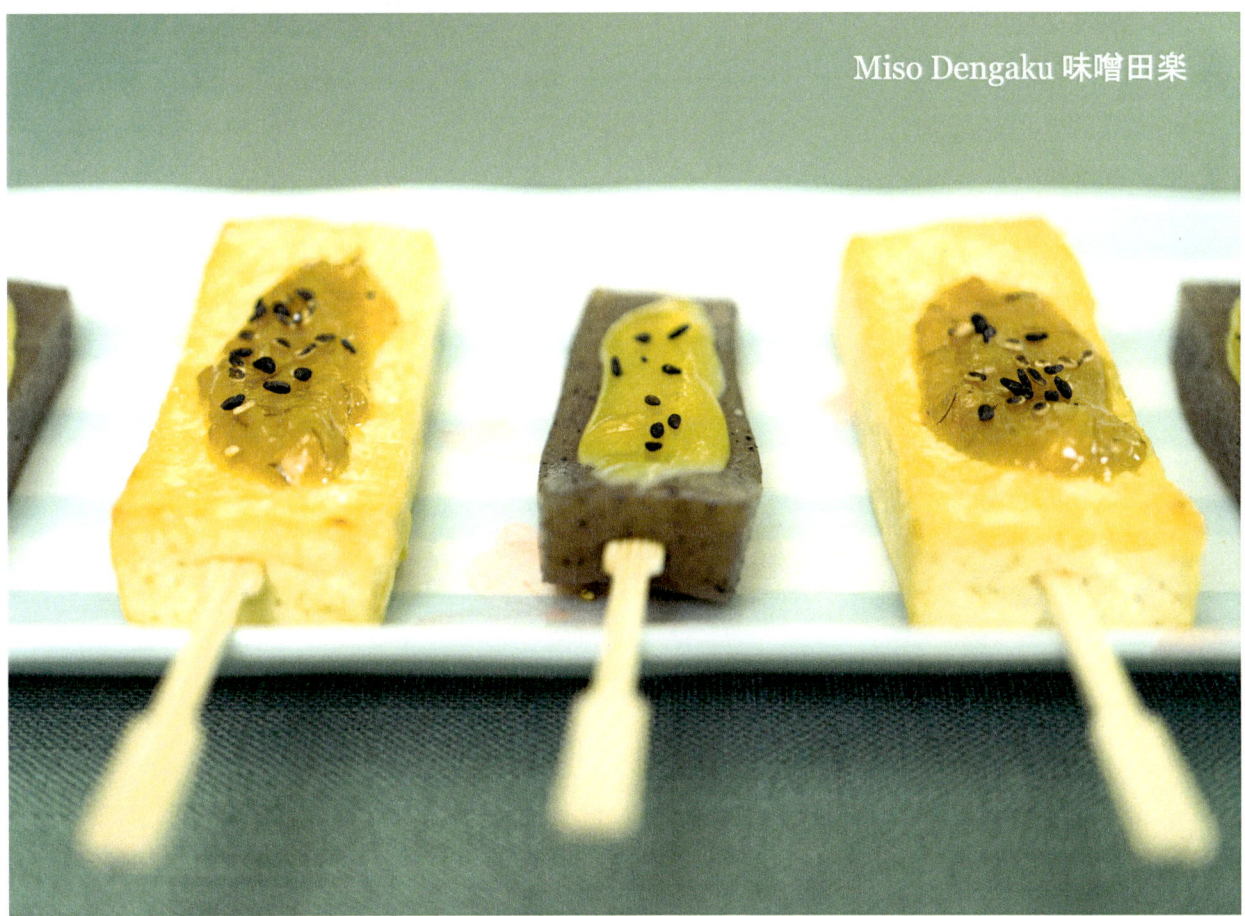

Miso Dengaku 味噌田楽

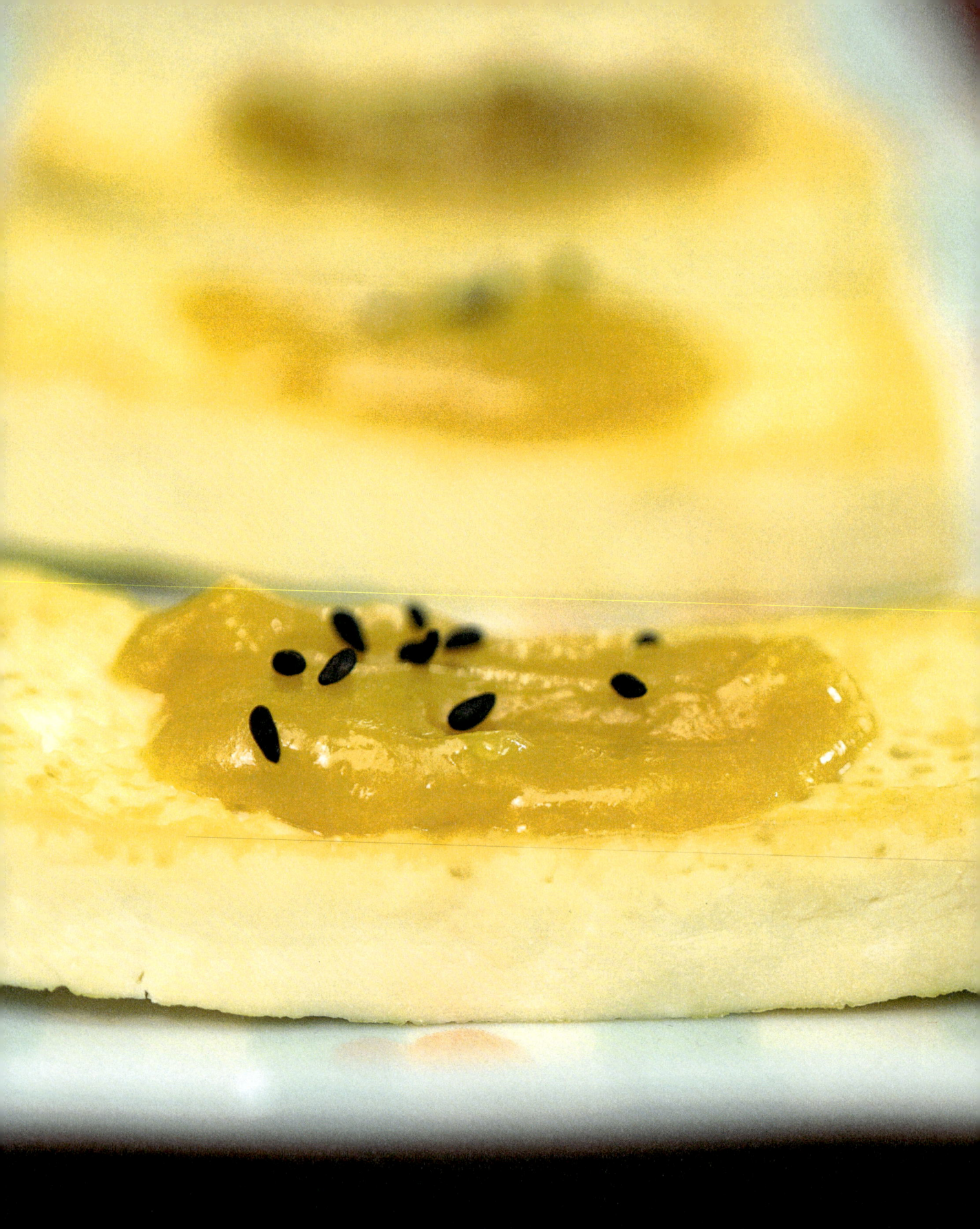

Miso Dengaku 味噌田楽

Miso dengaku 味噌田楽

Dengaku is rich and complex glaze that embodies the balance of sweet and savory. It took me several years to find a secret ingredient for my dengaku (egg yolk). Once you've had a taste... it might be hard to go back to one without it!

Serves 4

Ingredients

1 block firm tofu, cut into 2-3 in. long pieces
1 block konnyaku (9oz)

White miso dengaku
¼ cup white miso
1 egg yolk
2 Tbsp sake
2 Tbsp sugar
black sesame seeds, to garnish

Red miso dengaku
¼ cup red miso
1 egg yolk
2 Tbsp sake
2 Tbsp sugar
1 Tbsp mirin
1 tsp sesame oil
white sesame seeds, to garnish

Directions

1. Drain and rinse your konnyaku, cut konnyaku and tofu into small rectangles ½ in. thick.
2. Use a small pot with 1-2 cups water and boil the konnyaku for 2-3 minutes. Drain and set aside. *Boiling konnyaku helps to remove excess water and that unique odor it has out of the bag!*
4. Using the broiler in your oven, broil your tofu pieces for 2-3 minutes until they develop a light yellow/brown crust on top.
5. Meanwhile, use two sauce pans for each of the dengaku sauces, combine all the ingredients under white miso dengaku in one pan and red miso in another.
6. Heat dengaku sauces on low heat and cook for about 10 minutes. Mix frequently. The dengaku sauce is done once the clumps have disappeared and alcohol smell is gone.
7. Remove tofu from oven, skewer tofu and konnyaku and plate.
8. Use a spoon or spatula to spread 1-2 tsp dengaku sauce on each piece.
9. Garnish with sesame seeds and serve.

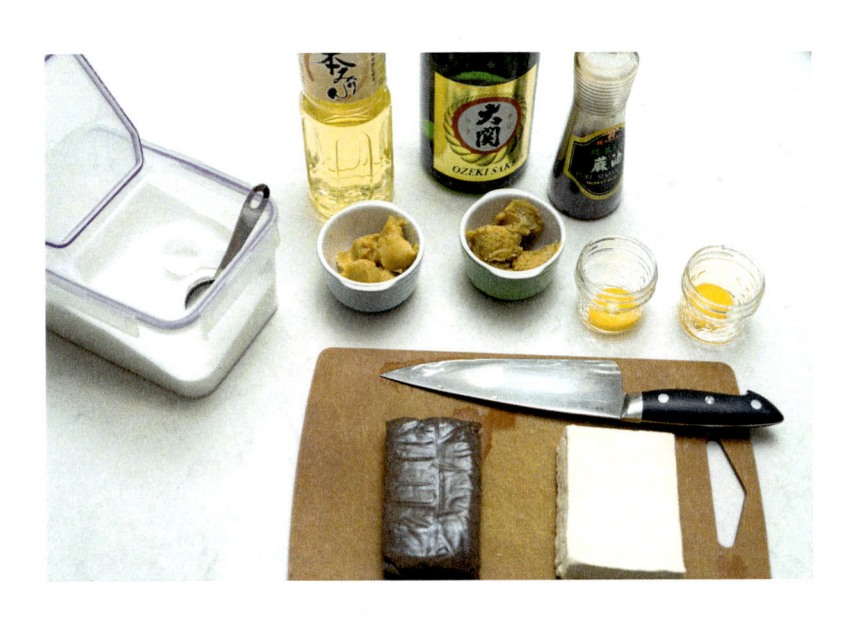

Ankakedoufu あんかけ豆腐

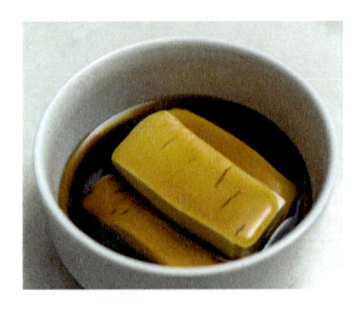

'Ankake' literally translated means 'sauce poured' or 'covered'. 'An' is a savory sauce typically made with dashi broth thickened using a starch like arrowroot flour (葛粉 - kuzoko) or potato starch (片栗粉 - katakuriko). For additional umami, gently cook your tofu in dashi stock for a few minutes before topping with the 'an'.

Serves 4

Ingredients

1 block soft tofu
2-3 in. square piece of konbu (5g) in ~2 cups water
2-3 stalks green onion, finely chopped
2-3 tsp ginger, grated
wasabi

For the an sauce
1 cup dashi, *recipe P. 23*
¼ cup soy sauce
½ Tbsp sugar
1 Tbsp potato starch, dissolved in 2 Tbsp water

Directions

1. Cut tofu into 6-8 large blocks.
2. Using a medium pot on low heat, add 1 cup water, konbu, and tofu. Allow to simmer (~15 min) while you prepare the other ingredients and make the an sauce.

For the an sauce
1. Using a small pot, combine the dashi stock, soy sauce, and sugar. Bring to a simmer.
2. Once the sugar has dissolved, add in the potato starch slurry and mix continuously for the first 15-20 seconds until the liquid has thickened evenly. Turn off heat.
3. Using a slotted spoon, remove the tofu blocks from the konbu stock, place in a small bowl.
4. Place tofu blocks on a bowl with rice or serving dish, pour over the thickened sauce.
5. Top with green onions, wasabi, and ginger.

Tips for working with potato starch (katakuriko):
- Always dissolve the potato starch in water, 1:1 or 1:2 ratio, never add direct or you'll get clumps
- Before adding, stir to redissolve starch if it has settled to the bottom
- Constantly stir while adding to the hot pot.
- Always ensure the solution you've added it to is very hot, if you don't notice thickening right away, your broth may not be hot enough. Continue heating on medium-high heat until you notice it starts to thicken.

Note- The konbu stock still has plenty of umami and can be reused for things like tounyuu nabe (recipe P. 84) or iridoufu (recipe P. 76)

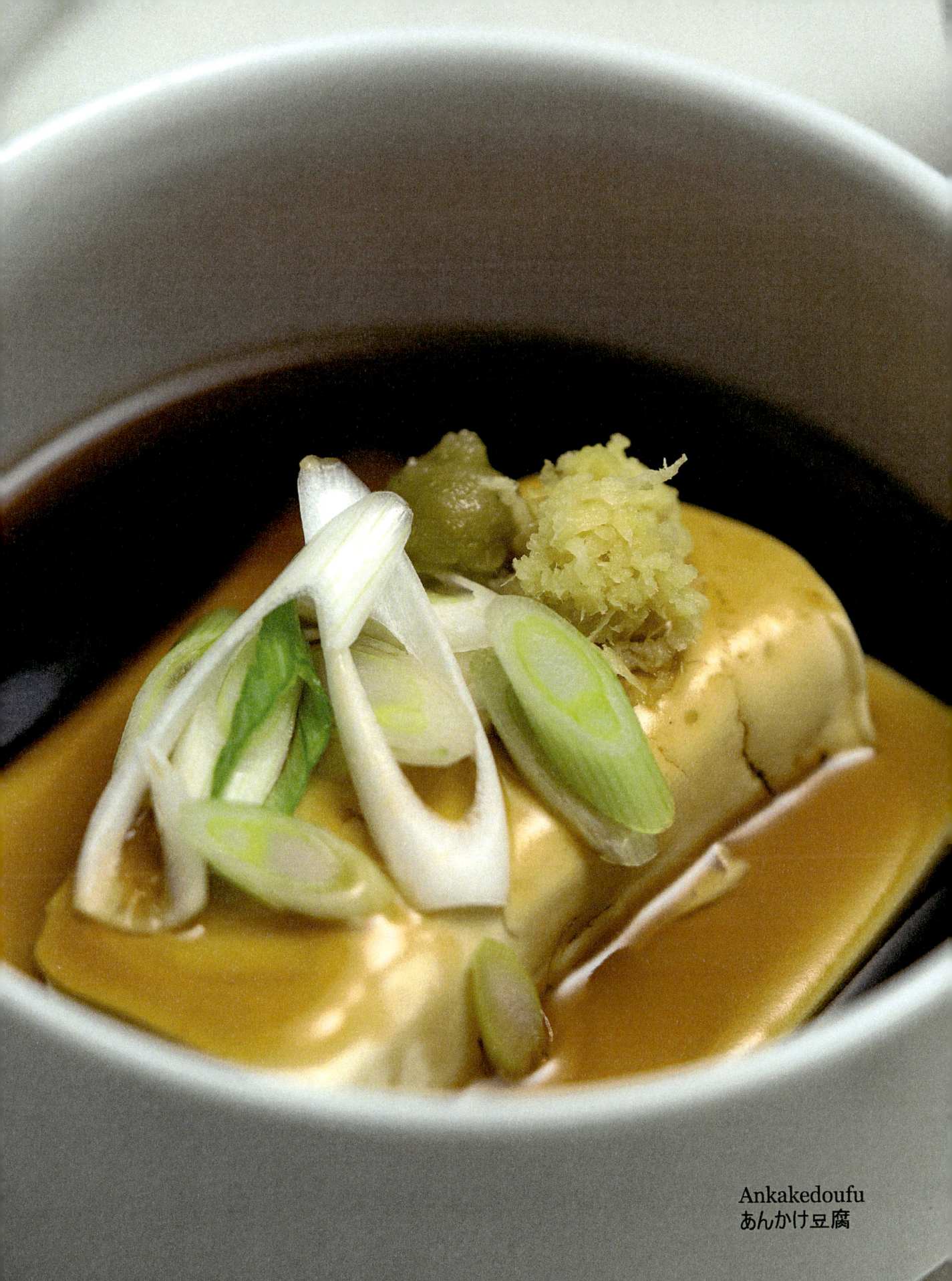

Ankakedoufu
あんかけ豆腐

Kinoko ankakedoufu
きのこあんかけ豆腐

I'm not sure there's any better combination of mushrooms with soy sauce, dashi, and mirin to make a thick and savory an sauce perfect for seasoning tofu. All I eat this with is rice, either as an appetizer or sometimes a complete meal!

Serves 4

Ingredients

1 block soft tofu
½ cup of enoki mushrooms (top part only)
1 cup shimeji mushrooms
½ cup shiitake mushrooms
1 cup dashi, *recipe P. 23*
dash of salt
1 tsp mirin
1 Tbsp soy sauce
1-2 green onions, sliced at an angle to garnish
1 Tbsp potato starch, dissolved in 2 Tbsp water

Directions

1. Prepare your mushrooms by rinsing and then cutting/breaking them apart. Set aside.
2. Using a medium saucepan, heat 1 cup dashi broth on medium heat.
3. Add a pinch of salt, mirin, soy sauce and mushrooms.
4. Bring to a simmer and cook at least 15-20 minutes partially covered.
5. Meanwhile, cut tofu into squares and set aside.
6. After mushrooms have cooked, add in tofu blocks and submerge in dashi mixture. Cook for another 10-15 minutes. *If not submerged try to rotate or flip halfway through.*
7. After tofu has cooked, use a slotted spoon or spatula to place into a serving bowl or plate.
8. Next add potato starch slurry to the pot (ensure it's well mixed prior to pouring). Mix thoroughly to avoid clumping. The mixture will thicken up right away.
9. Remove from heat and pour over tofu blocks, top with green onions, and serve!

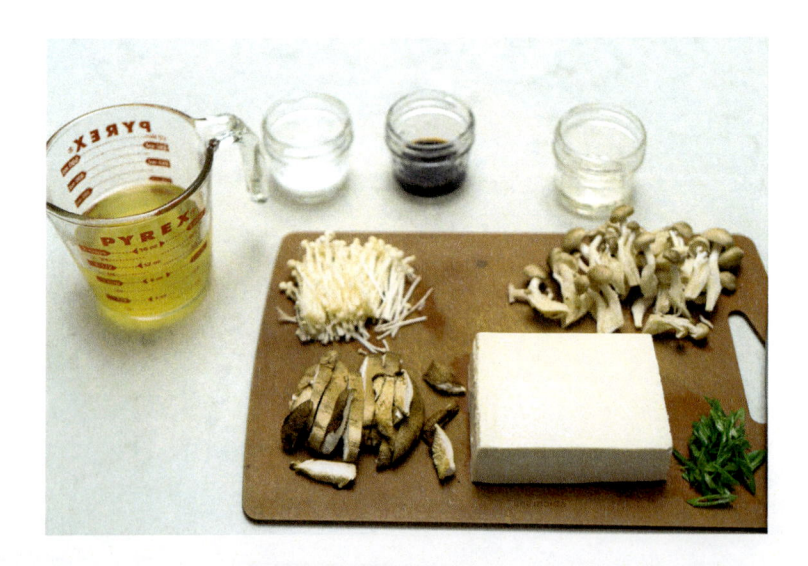

Kinoko Ankakedoufu
きのこあんかけ豆腐

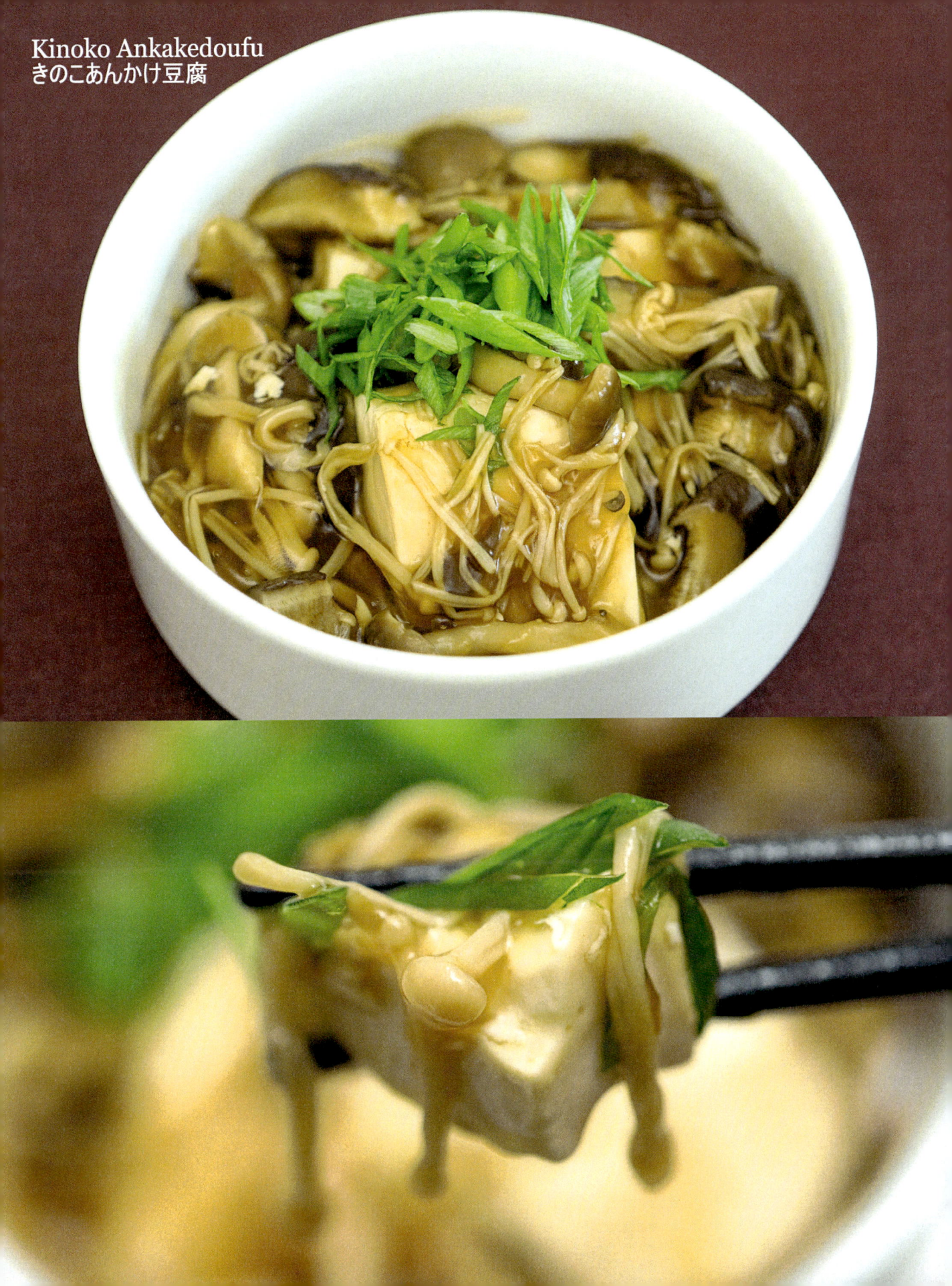

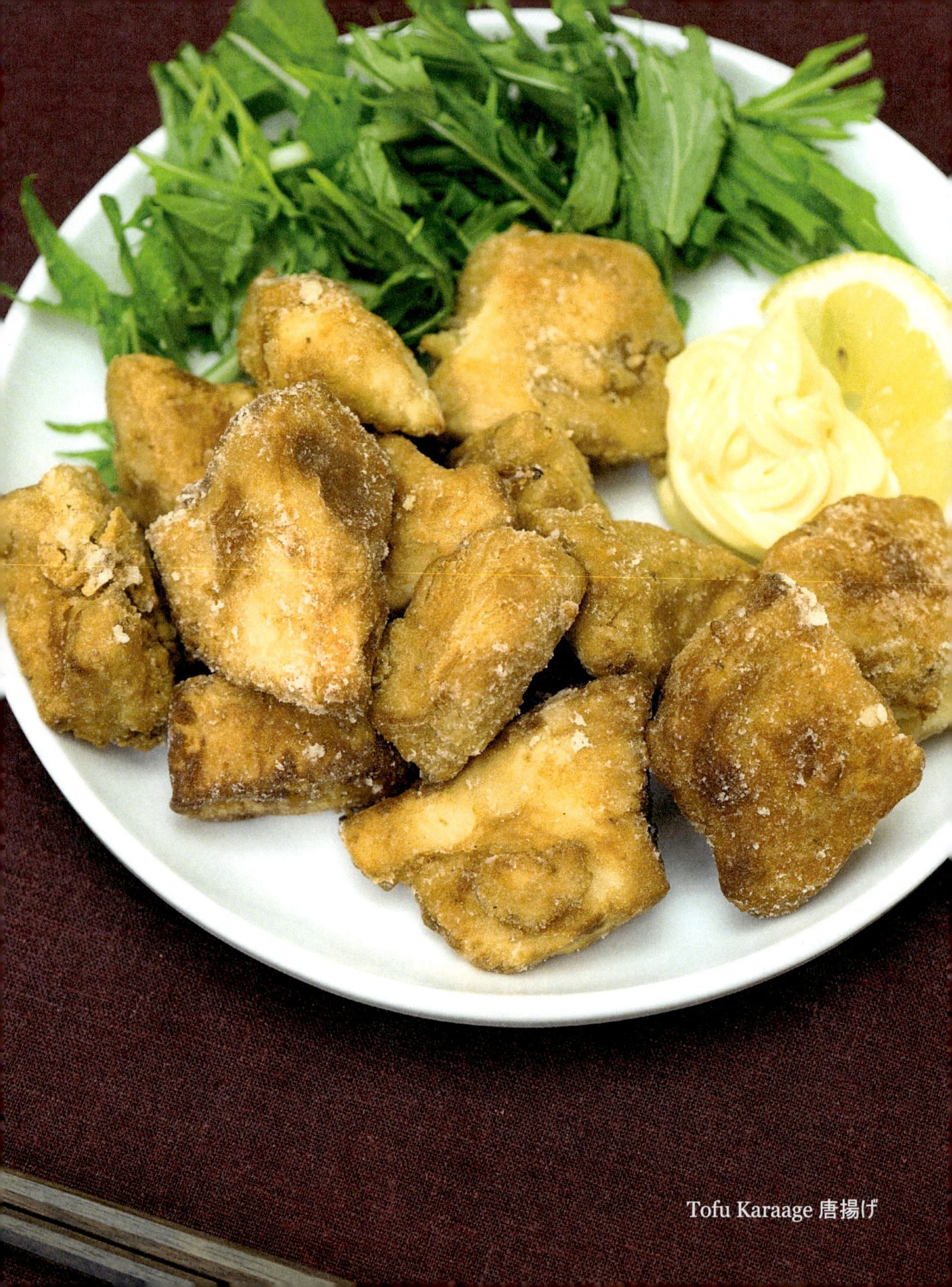

Tofu Karaage 唐揚げ

Tofu karaage 唐揚げ

Karaage is typically made with chicken that's marinated and then deep fried. However, this is the tofu version! I prefer soft tofu because I like the creamy texture, but if you want something firmer try it with firm tofu. You'll be pleasantly surprised at how similar this tastes to chicken karaage!

SERVES 4

INGREDIENTS

1 block soft tofu
1 cup canola oil for frying

For the marinade
6 Tbsp soy sauce
3 Tbsp sake
3 Tbsp mirin
1 Tbsp grated ginger
1 Tbsp crushed garlic
½ tsp chicken stock powder or paste
dash of white pepper
dash of sesame oil

For Dredging
¼ cup all-purpose flour
¼ cup potato starch
dash of salt and pepper

To serve
mizuna, thinly sliced cabbage, or baby greens; lemon wedges, Kewpie

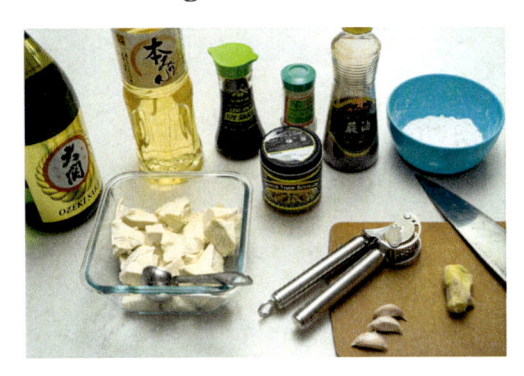

DIRECTIONS

1. Using your hands, gently tear tofu into bite size pieces and refrigerate uncovered over night. *This allows the outside to dry out slightly and makes it easier to dredge.*
2. The next day remove the tofu and pat dry with a paper towel.
3. Combine all the ingredients under marinade and add the tofu and allow to sit at least 30 minutes. If not completely submerged, rotate halfway through.
4. Heat a medium or large saucepan and add oil.
5. While the pan is heating, dredge the tofu blocks in the flour, potato starch, salt and pepper mixture.
6. Once oil is at 350 F, add the tofu blocks and fry until a light gold color - kitsuneiro (きつね色 - the color of a fox) roughly 2-3 minutes.
7. Remove from the pan and place on a paper towel lined plate to soak excess oil. Repeat with remaining pieces.
8. Serve with a wedge of lemon and Kewpie mayonnaise or yuzukosho.

Tip – craving the real thing? This is my go-to for the chicken version, so after making a block of tofu, there should be enough marinade leftover for 1/2 lb. of chicken. Marinate at least 30 minutes before frying. I'd love to hear which one you prefer more!

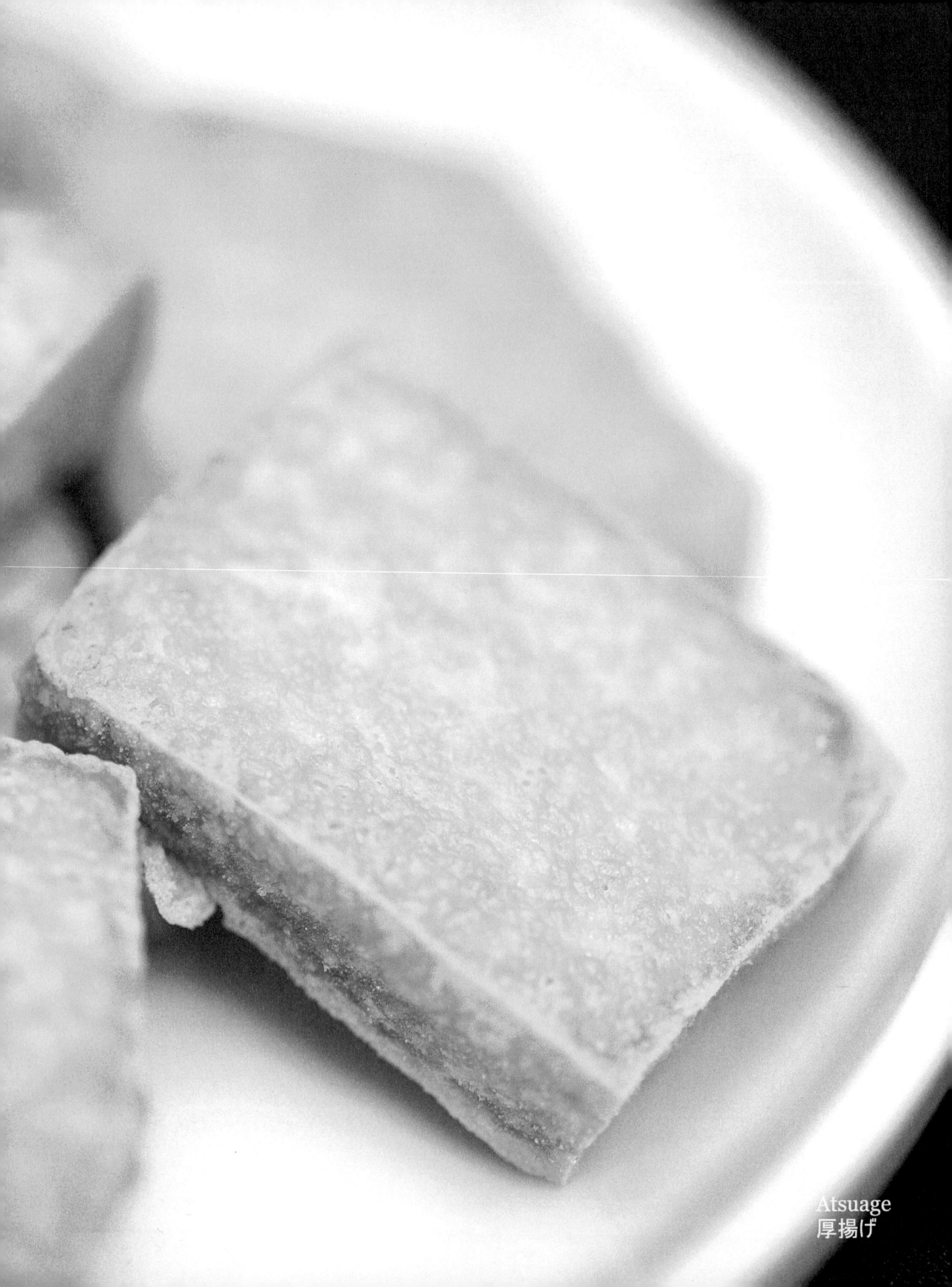

Atsuage
厚揚げ

Atsuage 厚揚げ

This is deep fried tofu. Ever had it? Not that easy to find, but that's probably a good thing. Otherwise, you might eat more than you should! Atsuage embodies what makes fried foods so delicious. Crunchy on the outside, soft and creamy on the inside. Fresh out of the fryer all you need is salt!

Serves 2-3

Ingredients

1 block firm or soft tofu
1 cup canola oil

Directions

1. Cut tofu into bite size squares or cubes, no more than ½ in. thick. Pat dry with a paper towel.
2. Bring oil to 350 degrees F in a small sauce pan. Once at temperature, gently add in tofu so that each piece is submerged.
3. Cook until color turns a light tan or as they say in Japanese kitsuneiro (きつね色 - the color of a fox) roughly 2-3 minutes.
4. Use a slotted spoon or skimmer to place on a paper towel plate to soak excess oil.
5. Serve immediately with soy sauce, grated daikon radish, momijioroshi (*recipe P. 86*), ponzu (*recipe P. 88*), nirajouyu (*recipe P. 89*) or plain salt!

Note- the blocks will get darker once removed from the oil. If you lose track of time, once they look like they might be turning a nice gold color around the edges (see below), that's when it's time to take them out!

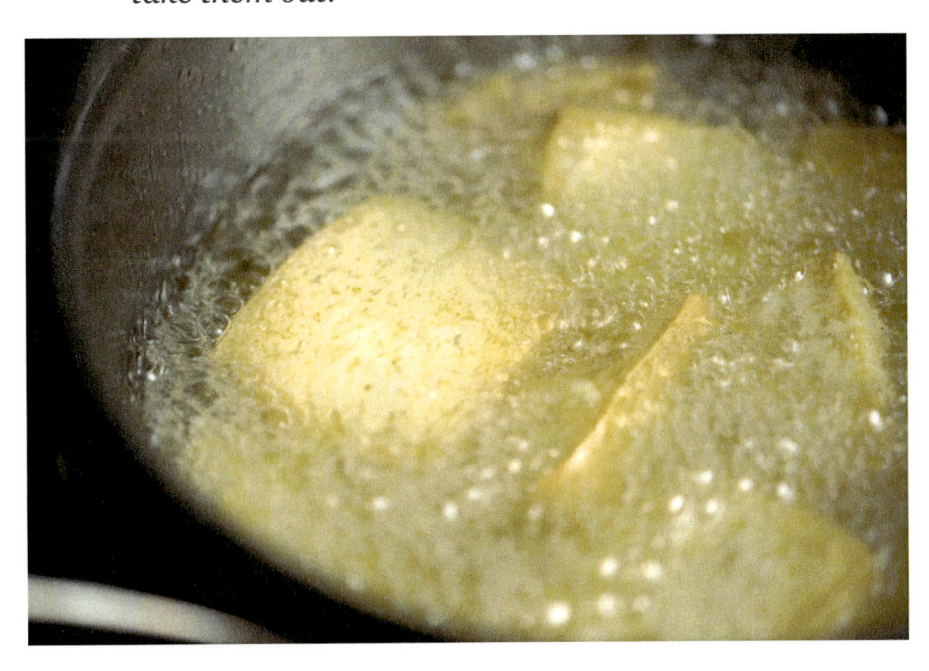

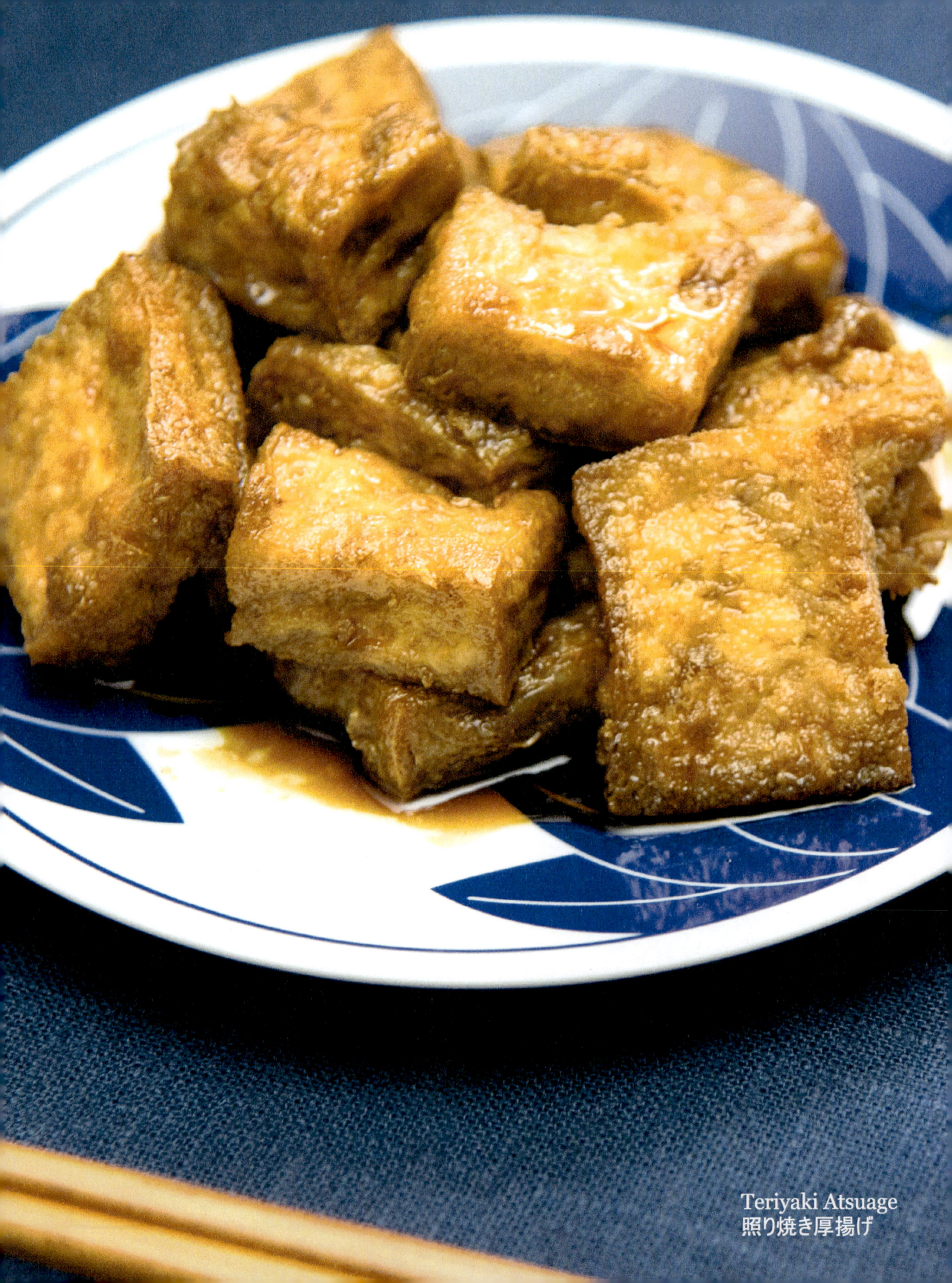

Teriyaki Atsuage
照り焼き厚揚げ

Teriyaki atsuage
照り焼き厚揚げ

This is deep fried tofu with teriyaki sauce. I don't normally make teriyaki since it's on the sweeter side of things, but if I do, I almost always make it with atsuage, yellowtail, or chicken. A good way to round out your teriyaki meal is by adding some sauteed vegetables like bell peppers, green onion or king mushroom!

SERVES 2-3

INGREDIENTS

1 tofu block worth of atsuage, *recipe P. 60*
4 Tbsp soy sauce
2 Tbsp mirin
1 Tbsp sugar
2-3 Tbsp extra-virgin olive oil

toppings- freshly ground sesame seeds, grated ginger, and/or chopped green onions

DIRECTIONS

1. If working with one large block of atsuage, cut into bite size pieces, or 1 in. blocks.
2. Pat dry with a paper towel to soak excess oil.
3. Mix the ingredients for the teriyaki sauce in a small mixing bowl and set aside.
4. Heat a medium or large skillet on medium heat with extra-virgin olive oil. When shimmering add the atsuage and cook for 1 minute to heat through.
5. Add the teriyaki sauce to the atsuage and quickly stir to ensure each piece is coated.
6. Once the sauce has reduced and thickened (to a ketchup like consistency) remove from heat and serve.
7. Garnish with freshly ground sesame seeds, grated ginger, and/or green onions.

Optional step 1- to cut down on the oil you eat, remove excess oil from atsuage by boiling in hot water for 1-2 minutes. Pat dry.
Optional step 2- lightly coat each piece with potato or corn starch for an extra sticky and saucy teriyaki that will cling to the atsuage.

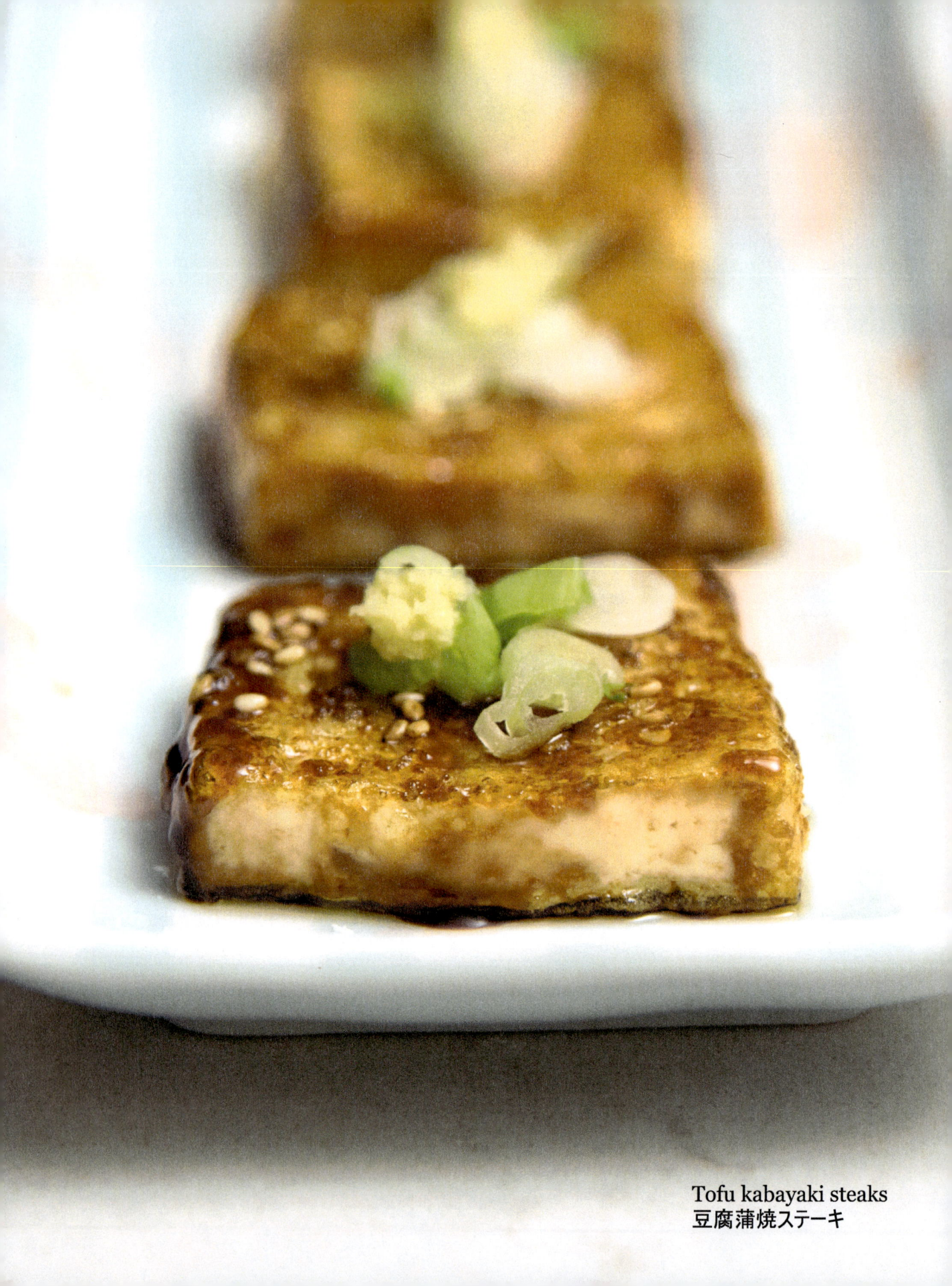

Tofu kabayaki steaks
豆腐蒲焼ステーキ

Tofu kabayaki steaks
豆腐蒲焼ステーキ

Kabayaki is a popular way to season and cook eel. The real thing is extremely delicious and full of fat, flavor, and umami. Tofu may not have all the fat and flavor of eel, but is an excellent vehicle for this tasty kabayaki sauce. And no, as much as I'd love to say it, it doesn't come close to the real thing. It's different and delicious in own unique tofu-ey way!

SERVES 4

INGREDIENTS

1 block firm tofu
3-4 Tbsp potato starch
ginger, freshly grated
1-2 green onions, finely chopped
1 Tbsp sesame seeds, toasted
extra-virgin olive oil for pan-frying

Kabayaki sauce
3 Tbsp soy sauce
2 Tbsp mirin
2-4 drops honey
1 Tbsp sake
1-2 tsp grated ginger with juice

toppings- chopped green onion, grated ginger, sansho pepper

DIRECTIONS

First make the sauce
1. Mix all ingredients in a small mixing bowl or jar. Set aside.

For the steaks
1. Microwave the tofu with a paper towel in a bowl for 2 minutes and 30 seconds.
2. Cut tofu into flat 1 in. squares, ½ in. thick.
3. Pat dry and coat lightly on all sides with potato starch.
4. Using medium heat, add 2-3 Tbsp extra-virgin olive oil to a large skillet and when shimmering, add the tofu squares.
5. Pan-fry both sides until they've turned a light gold, roughly 2-3 minutes per side.
6. Once the second side has lightly browned, turn heat to medium-low and add the kabayaki sauce to the pan and cook until thickened. About 1 minute.
7. Once each square is thoroughly coated, top with desired garnishes, and serve.

Tips - you may need to do this in two batches depending on how big your pan is. Reserve half of the sauce for the other half of the tofu block.
- If you're out of potato starch, use corn starch or all-purpose flour. All-purpose flour will give a nice coating, but may not allow the sauce to stick as well as with starch.
- If you really enjoy the flavor of sesame oil, consider frying in a 1:1 mixture of sesame to olive oil or 100% sesame oil!

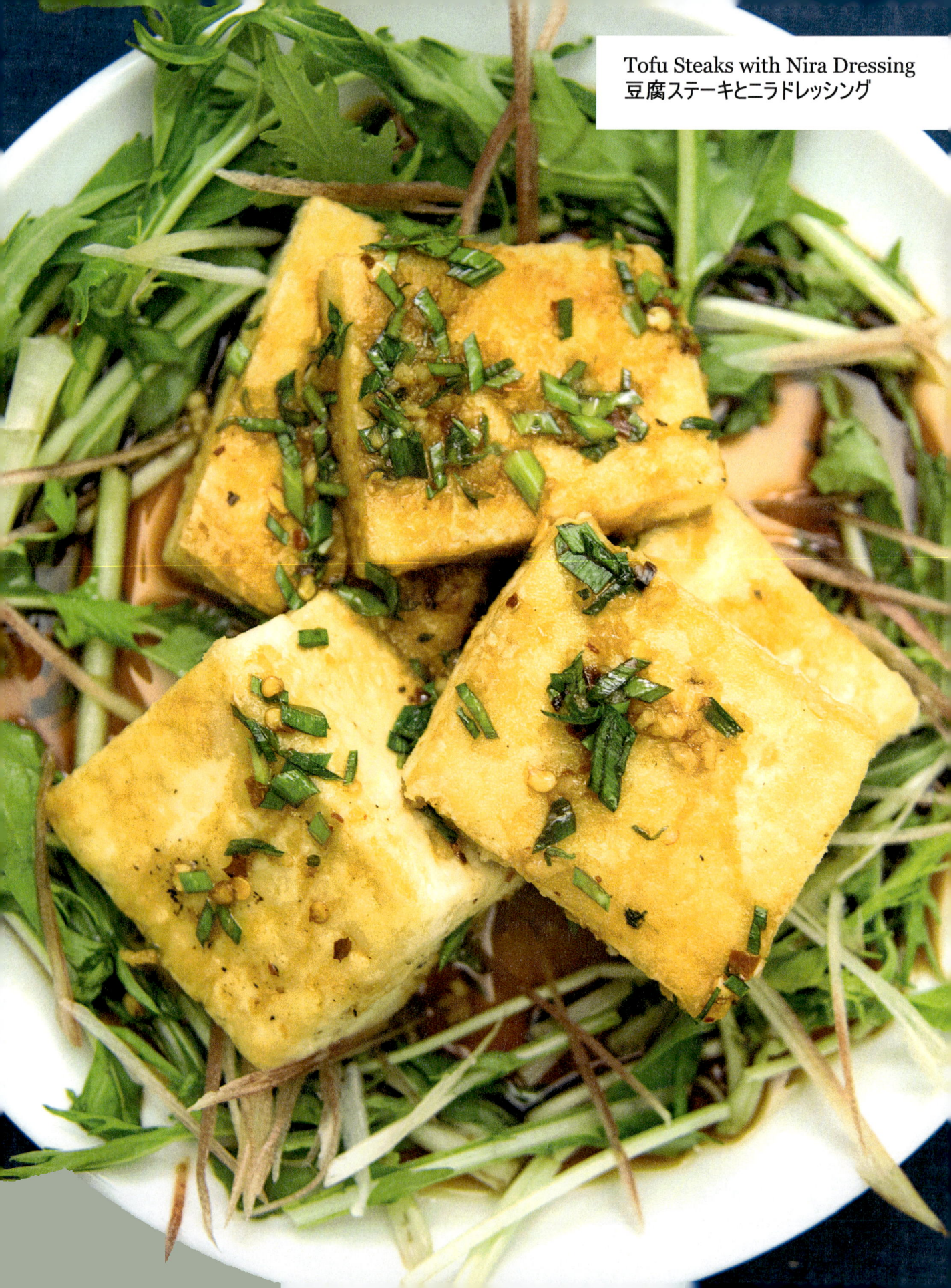

Tofu Steaks with Nira Dressing
豆腐ステーキとニラドレッシング

Tofu steaks with nira dressing
豆腐ステーキとニラドレッシング

A simple way to season your tofu steaks. Reminiscent of nirajouyu ニラ醤油, but with a little vinegar for acidity and added depth! These steaks are right at home on a bed of greens and myoga, if you can find it. If not, red onion will add the color and another layer of flavor that'll make this look and taste just as delicious!

SERVES 4

INGREDIENTS

1 block firm tofu
all-purpose flour, as needed for coating
2 Tbsp extra-virgin olive oil
1 cup mixed baby greens and/or mizuna, chopped
¼ cup myoga or red onion, thinly sliced
1-2 tsp toasted sesame seeds to garnish

For the dressing
2 Tbsp soy sauce
2 Tbsp rice vinegar
2 tsp mirin
1 clove garlic, crushed
1 tsp sesame oil
dash of red pepper flakes
2-3 tsp nira, finely chopped

optional toppings—chopped green onions, ichimi or shichimi red pepper, red pepper flakes

DIRECTIONS

1. Cut tofu into 8 squares or bite size pieces.
2. Using a large sauté pan on medium heat add 2 Tbsp olive oil.
3. Cover tofu pieces lightly with all purpose flour and add to the pan.
4. Pan-fry on both sides until slightly browned and remove from heat.
5. Place tofu steaks over a bed of mixed baby greens or mizuna and myoga strips (or thinly sliced red onion).
6. Top with the dressing and serve!

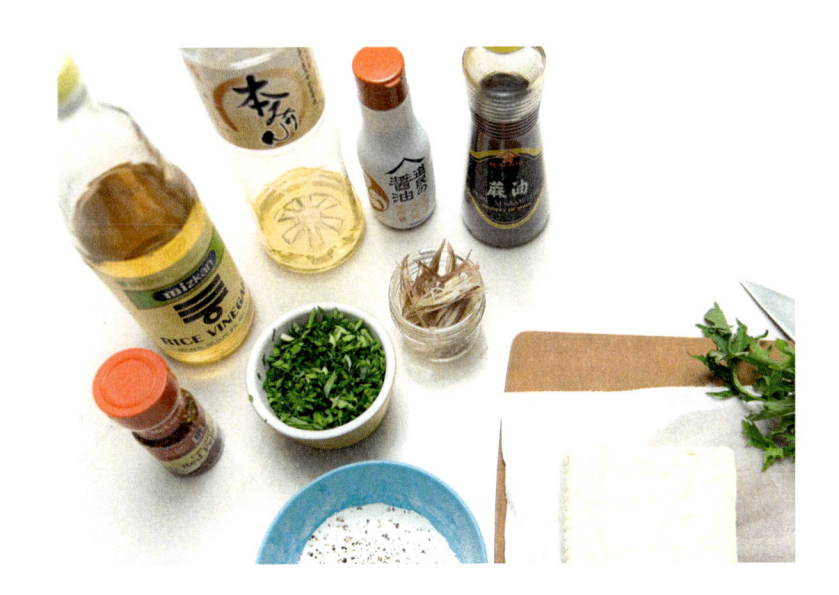

Pan Fried tofu steaks with nira dressing

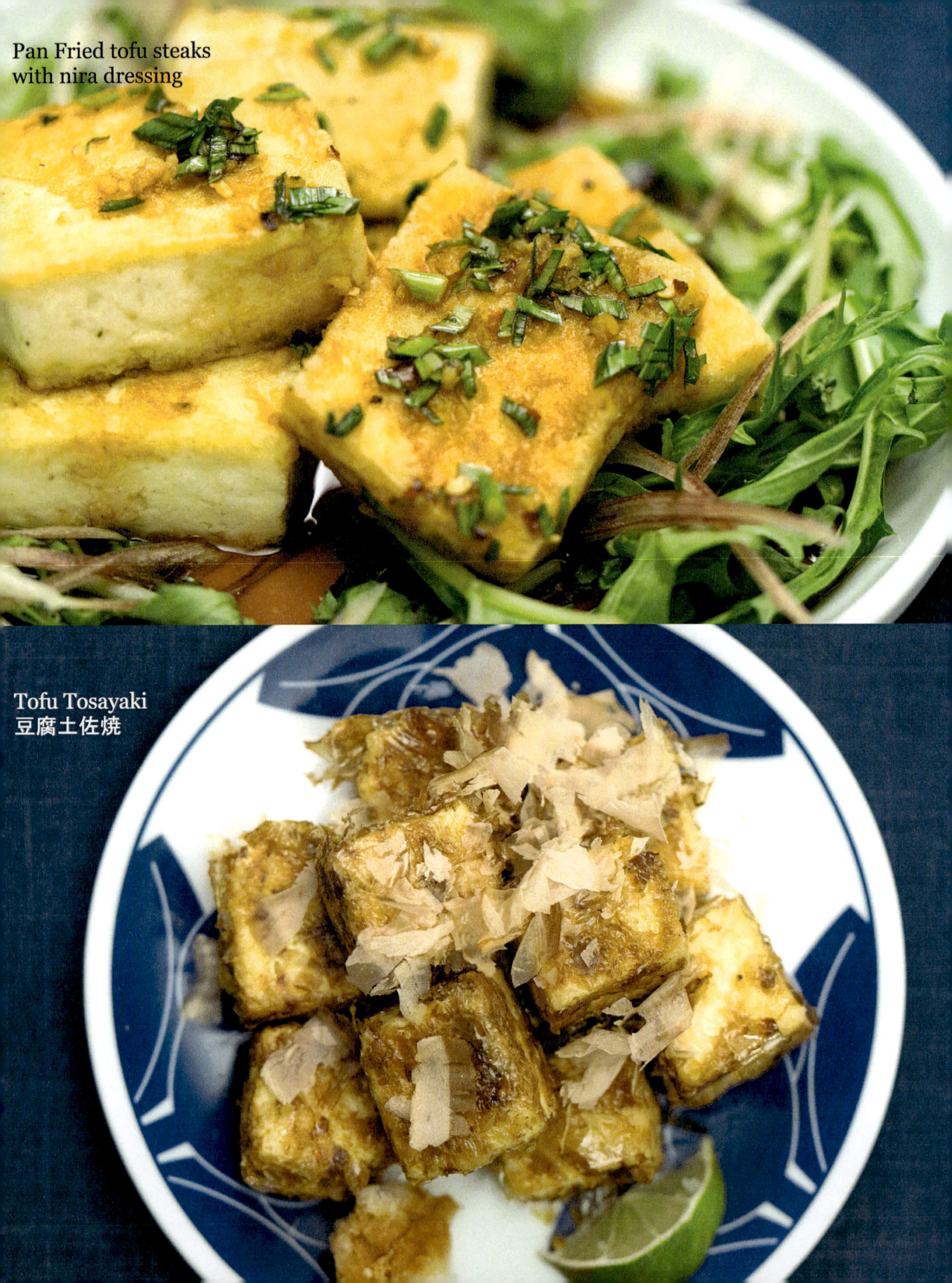

Tofu Tosayaki
豆腐土佐焼

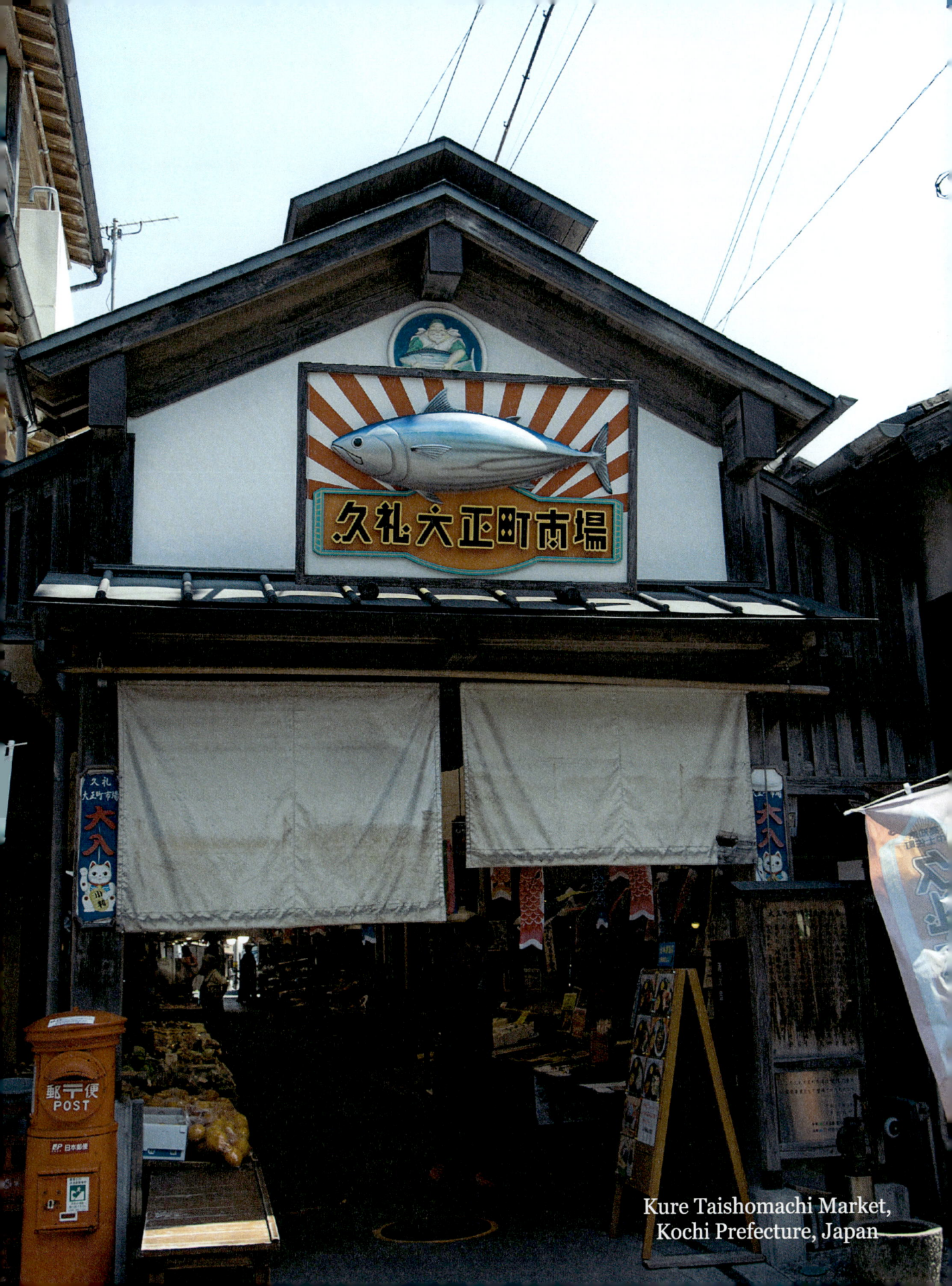

Kure Taishomachi Market,
Kochi Prefecture, Japan

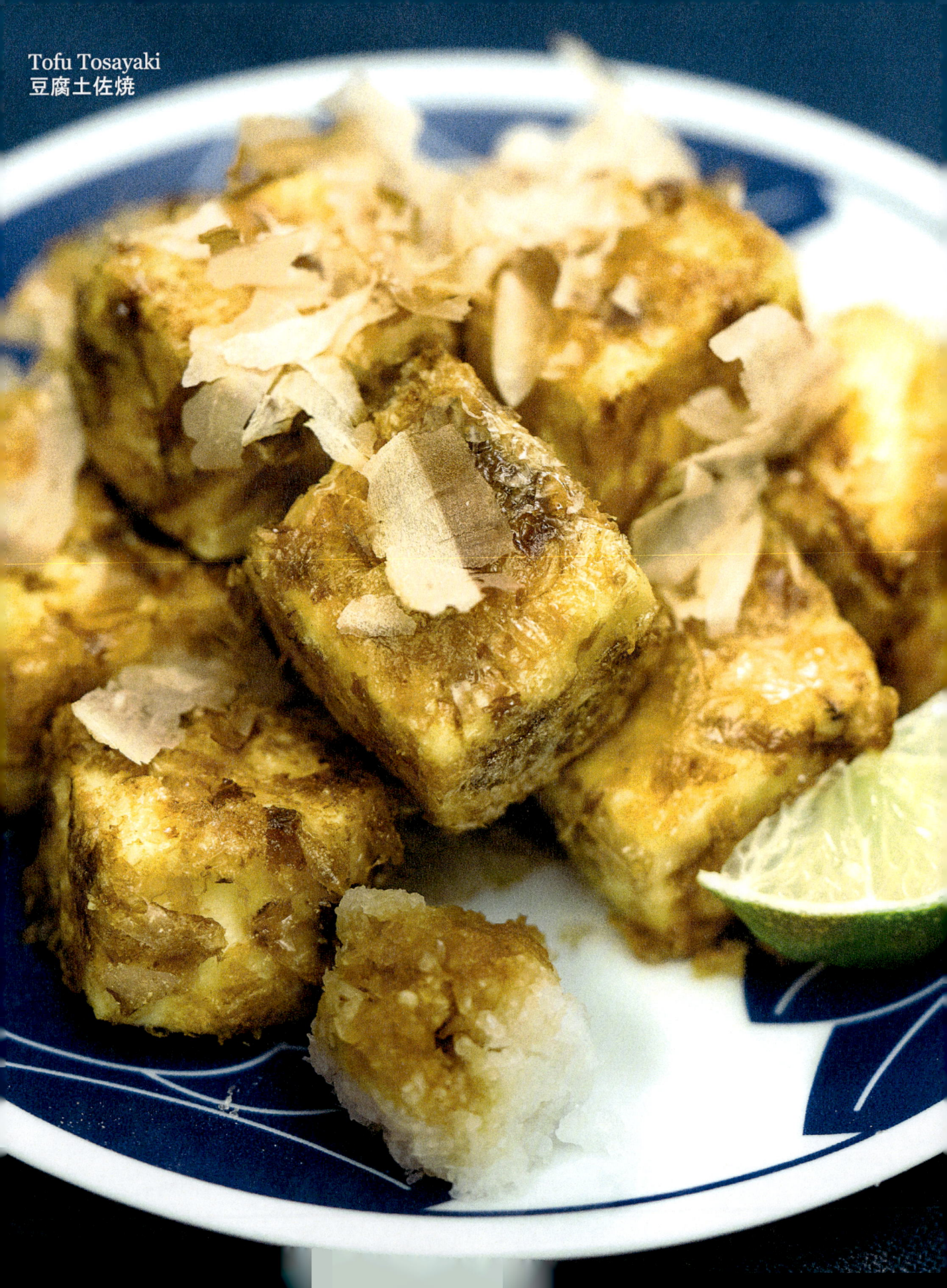

Tofu Tosayaki
豆腐土佐焼

Tofu tosayaki 豆腐土佐焼 (katsuobushi crusted tofu)

Tosa is a famous town and region in Shikoku. This area of Shikoku is famous for katsuobushi (bonito). More specifically, wara no tataki (藁のタタキ straw seared bonito). This dish reminds me of my visits to Shikoku and eating wara no tataki!

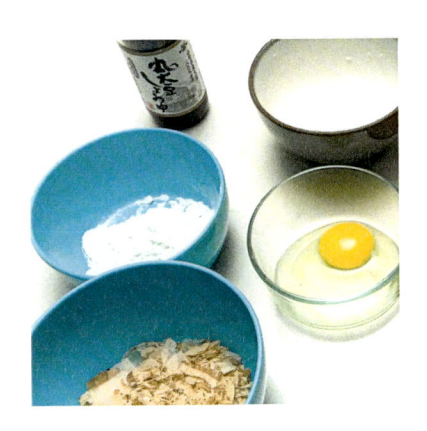

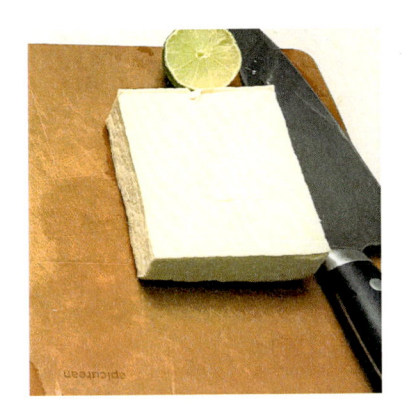

SERVES 4

INGREDIENTS

1 block soft tofu
all-purpose flour, for dredging
1 egg, whisked
¾ cup katsuobushi flakes, more as needed
extra-virgin olive oil for pan frying

Grated daikon, ¼ cup, excess water removed
Lime, soy sauce or ponzu

Optional- chopped green onions, grated ginger

DIRECTIONS

1. Cut tofu into bite size cubes.
2. First coat the tofu pieces in flour, then egg, then katsuobushi flakes.
3. Using medium heat, add 1-2 Tbsps extra-virgin olive oil to a large sauté pan and when shimmering add the tofu pieces.
4. Cook each side until slightly browned and rotate until all sides are browned.
5. Once cooked set on a plate, serve with grated daikon radish, lime, and soy sauce or ponzu (*recipe P. 88*)

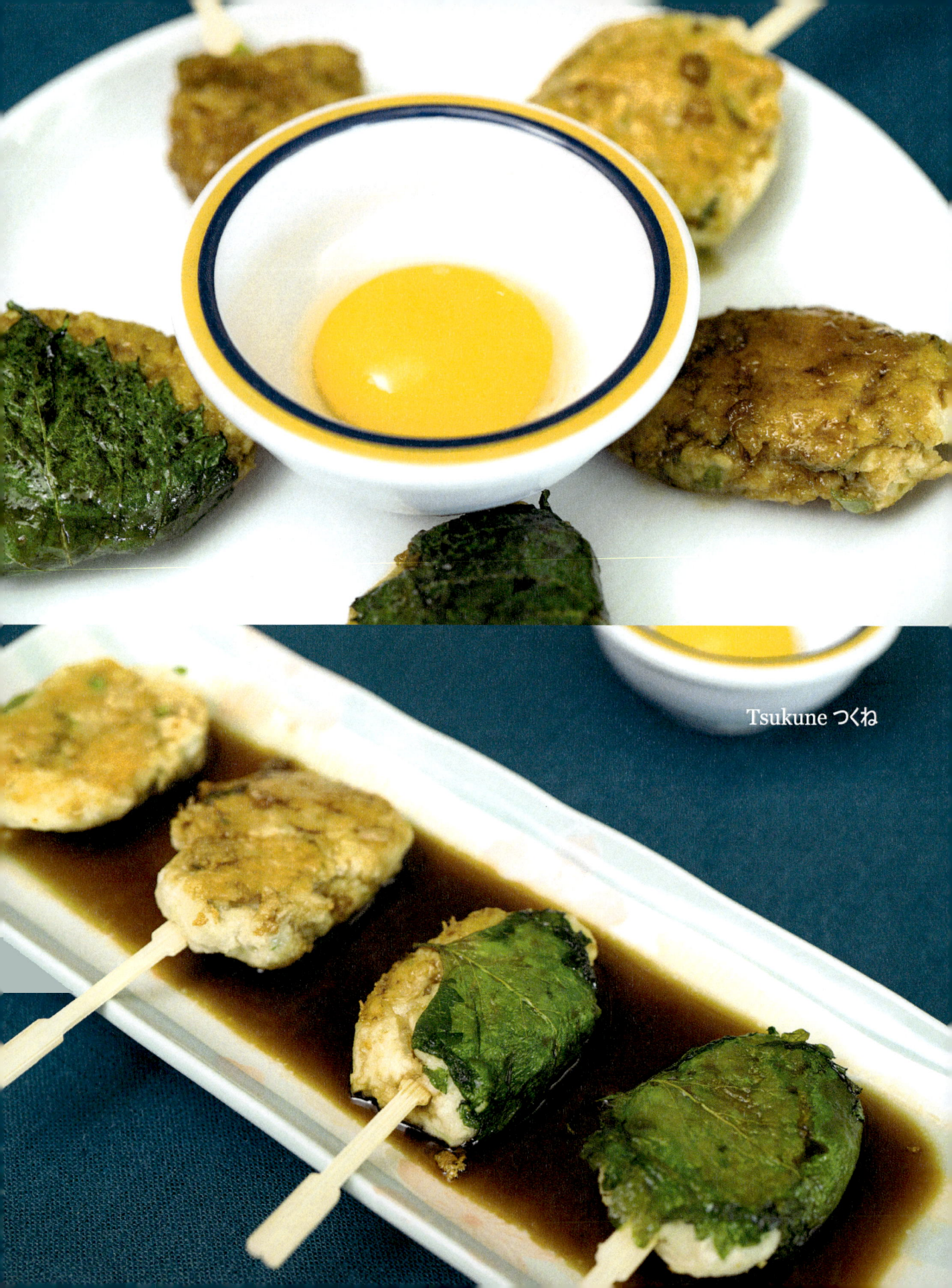

Tsukune つくね

Tsukune つくね

Tsukune reminds me of eating at yakitoriya (焼き鳥屋 - yakitori specialty) shops in Japan. It's one of the best things you can pair with alcohol. It's fatty, savory, and won't fill you up! Usually it's made with chicken, but here we're adding in a little tofu and topping it with a super magical and delicious kabayaki sauce!

SERVES 3-4

Ingredients

4 oz renkon, grated
4 oz firm tofu
½ lb. ground chicken
1 stalk green onion, finely chopped
2 tsp grated ginger
2 Tbsp potato starch
Dash of salt
Sesame oil
optional - raw egg yolk

For the sauce
¼ cup sake
¼ cup mirin
¼ cup soy sauce

Directions

1. First mix the ingredients under sauce in a small bowl and set aside.
2. Grate renkon and combine with tofu in a food processor and process until smooth.
3. Using a large bowl, combine chicken, ginger, green onions, the processed renkon/tofu, and potato starch. Use a spatula to mix thoroughly.
4. Using oiled hands form flat popsicle like patties about 1 in. wide to 2-3 in. long and set aside.
5. Using a large pan, heat 2-3 Tbsps of sesame oil on medium heat and pan-fry the patties until lightly browned, then flip.
6. As you cook the tsukune patties, place the sauce ingredients in a small saucepan and heat on medium heat. Cook and allow to thicken (~10 minutes) then remove from heat.
6. After flipping over the tsukune and browning the second side, remove from pan and set aside.
7. Use small skewers to pierce each patty from one end, serve with sauce and rice!

Notes - you can cook the kabayaki sauce with the tsukune patties as well, the sauce may be absorbed a bit better, but it takes a little longer.
- eating raw egg yolk may increase your risk of foodborne illness, eat at your own risk!

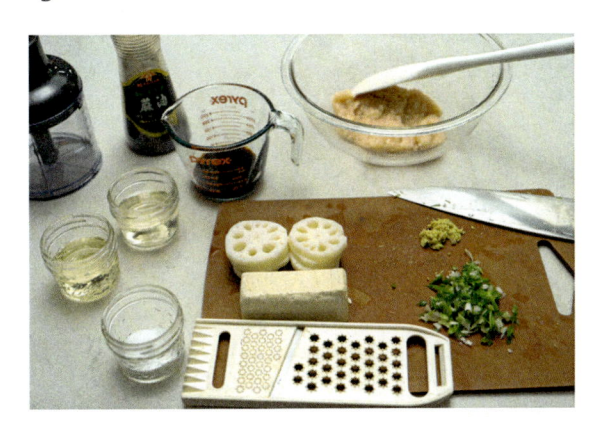

Main Dishes

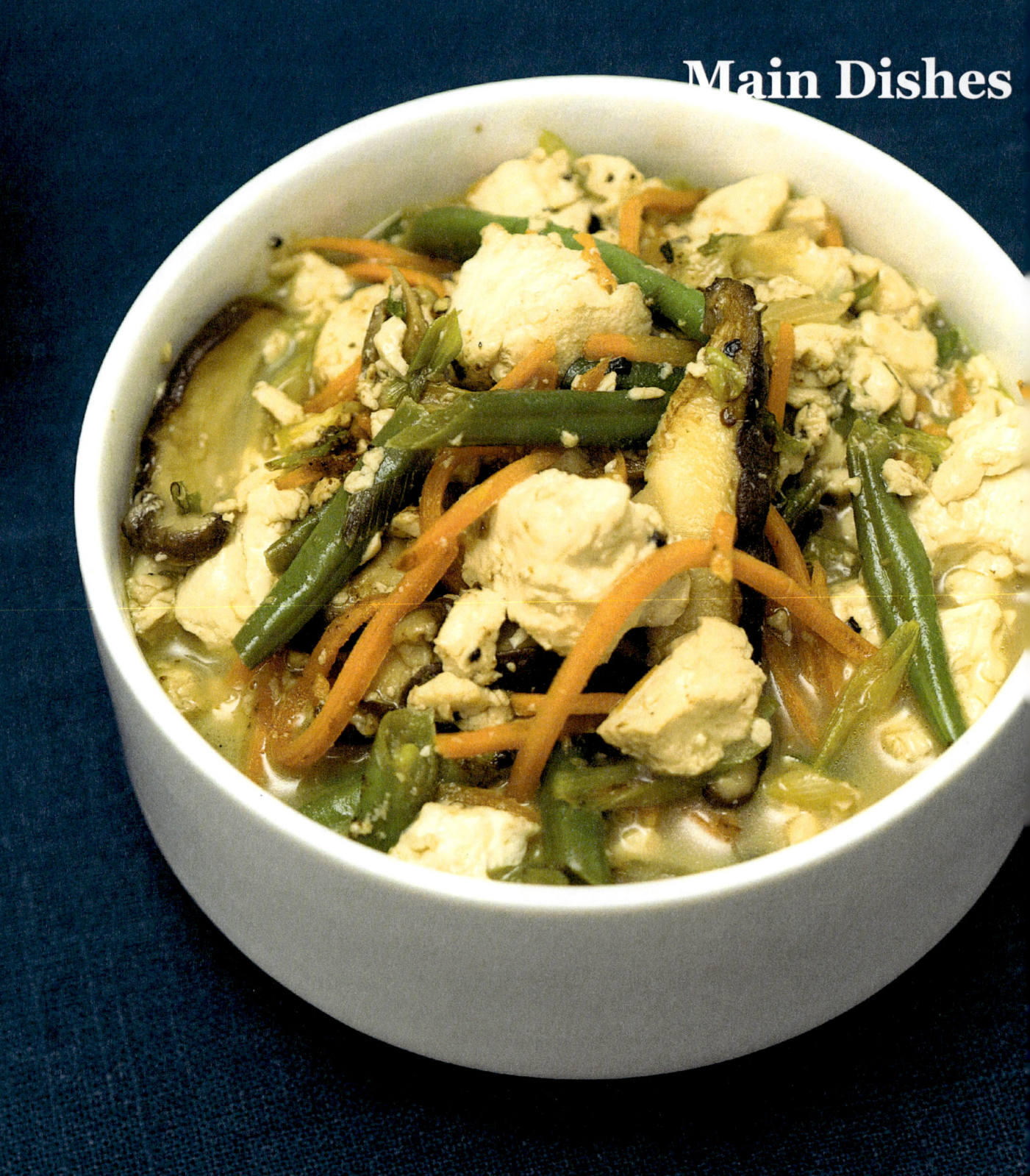

Iridoufu 煎り豆腐

Tounyuu nabe 豆腐豆乳鍋

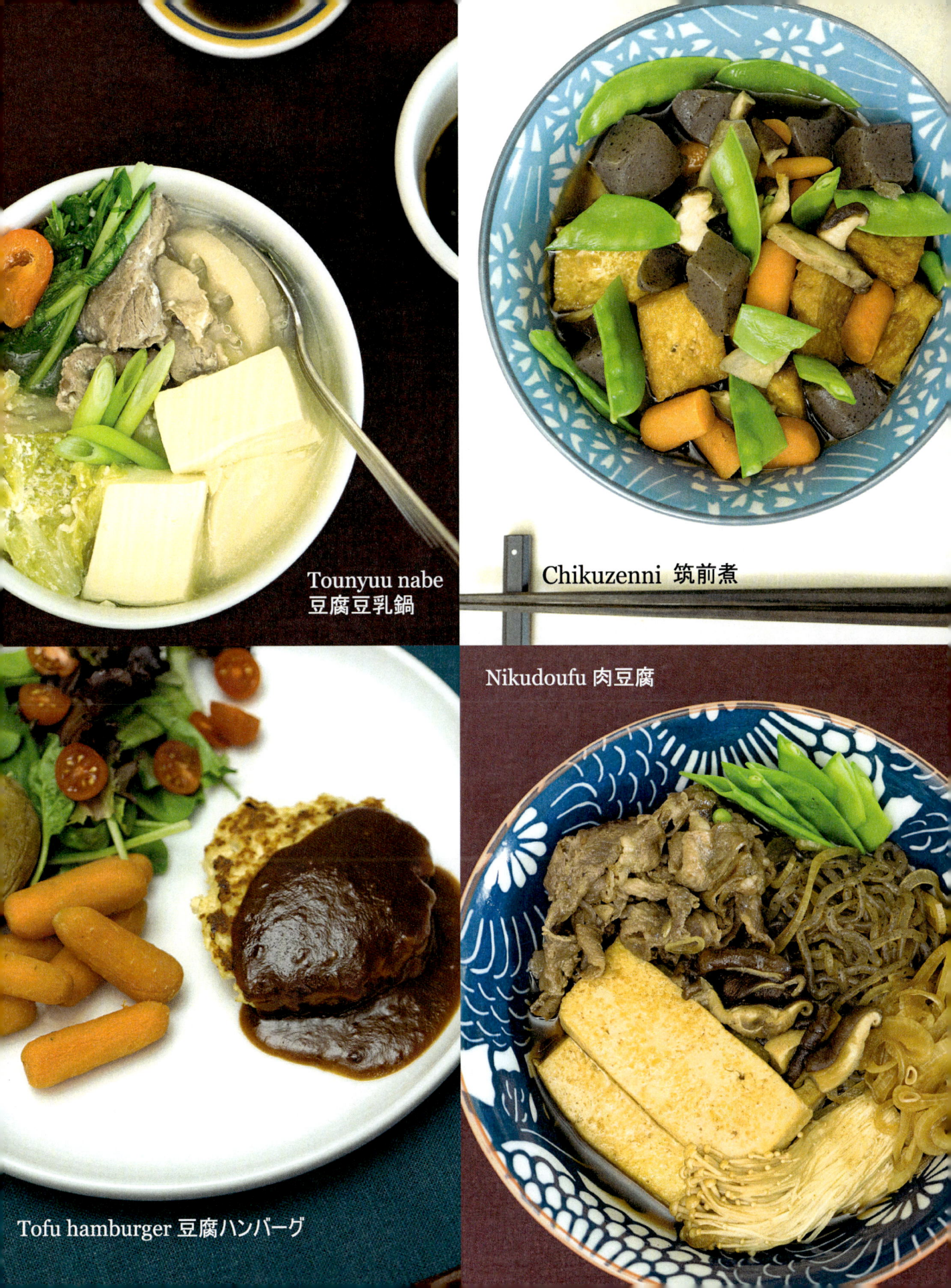

Chikuzenni 筑前煮

Tofu hamburger 豆腐ハンバーグ

Nikudoufu 肉豆腐

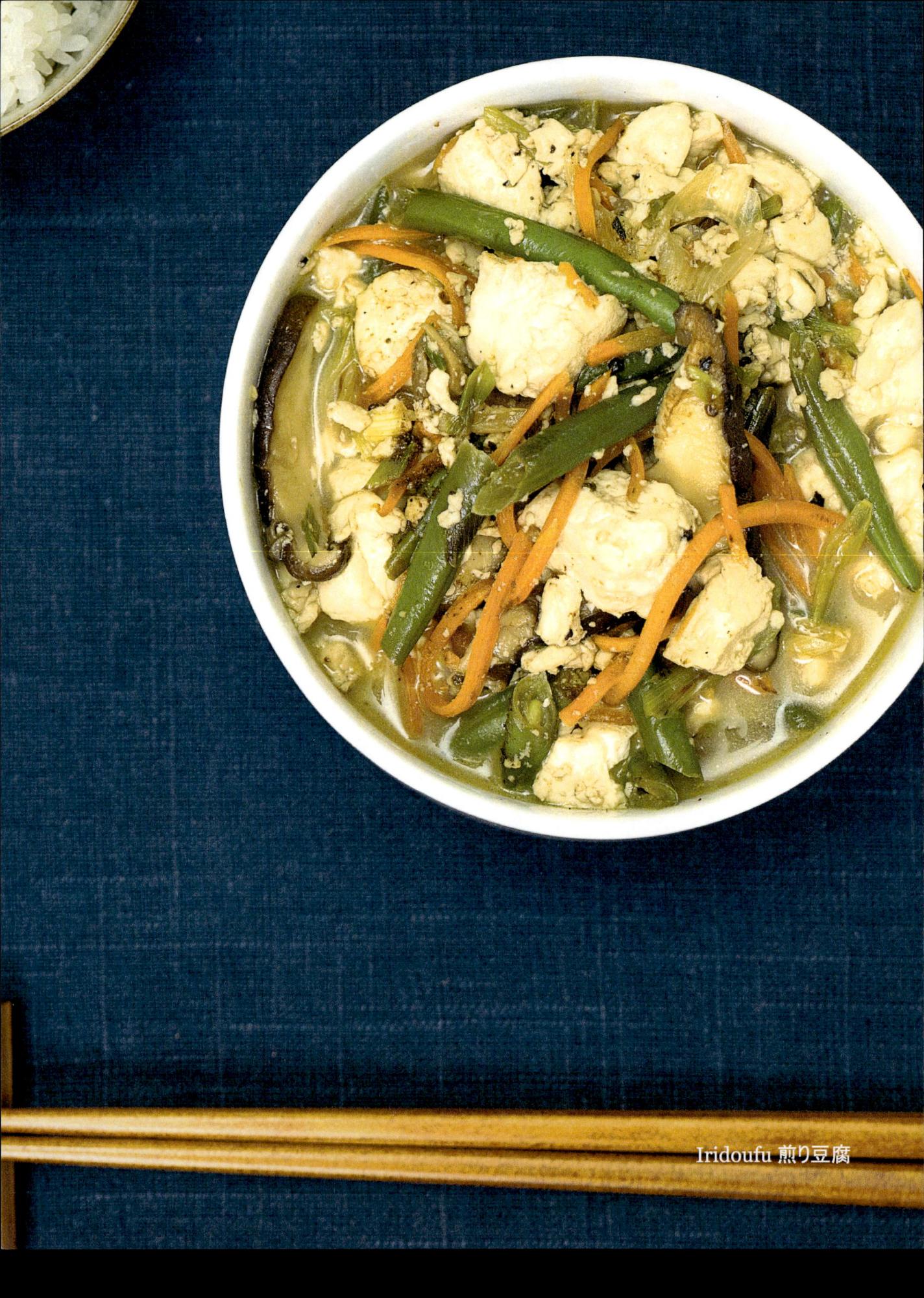

Iridoufu 煎り豆腐

Iridoufu 煎り豆腐

Iridoufu is essentially a tofu scramble. You can add all the things you normally might add to an omelette or scrambled egg, and you can even include eggs too. The texture is almost like egg whites, but unlike egg whites, it'll never be rubbery. This version calls for konbu dashi, which adds a good base flavor that'll have you eating this iridoufu again and again!

Serves 4

Ingredients

1 block soft tofu
1 cup green beans, trimmed
1 cup carrots, shredded
½ cup green onions, chopped
2-3 shiitake mushrooms, sliced
1 Tbsp sesame oil
½-1 Tbsp extra-virgin olive oil
½ cup konbu dashi, *recipe P. 21*
2 Tbsp light soy sauce
2 Tbsp mirin
white pepper and black pepper, to taste

Directions

1. Microwave the tofu for 2 minutes. Meanwhile, prepare and chop vegetables.
2. Add extra-virgin olive oil and sesame oil to pan and cook carrots for 1-2 minutes.
3. Add in the green beans then the mushrooms and cook for 2-3 minutes.
4. Add in the dashi stock, mirin, and soy sauce. Add a dash of white and black pepper if desired.
5. Reduce liquid to desired consistency or until heated through.
6. Serve with rice.

Note - try making this with regular dashi for an equally tasty iridoufu!

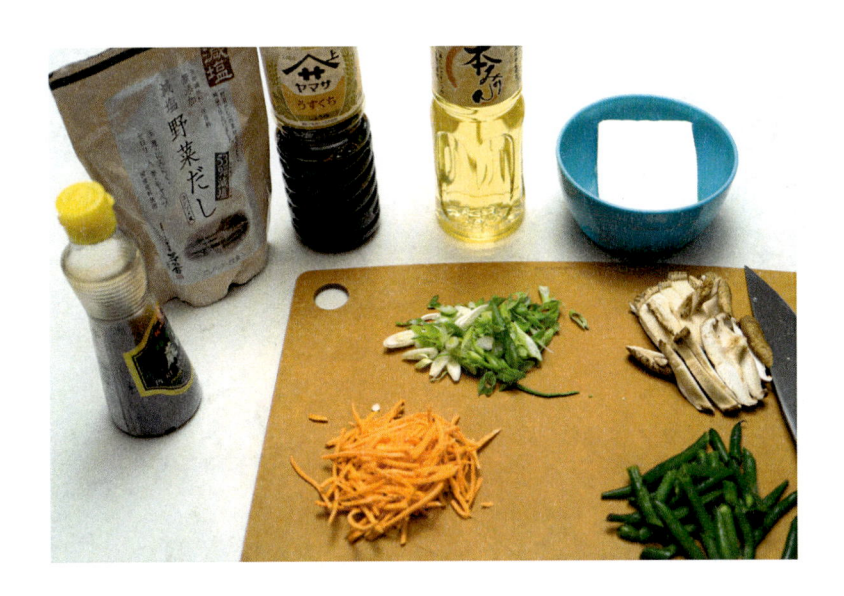

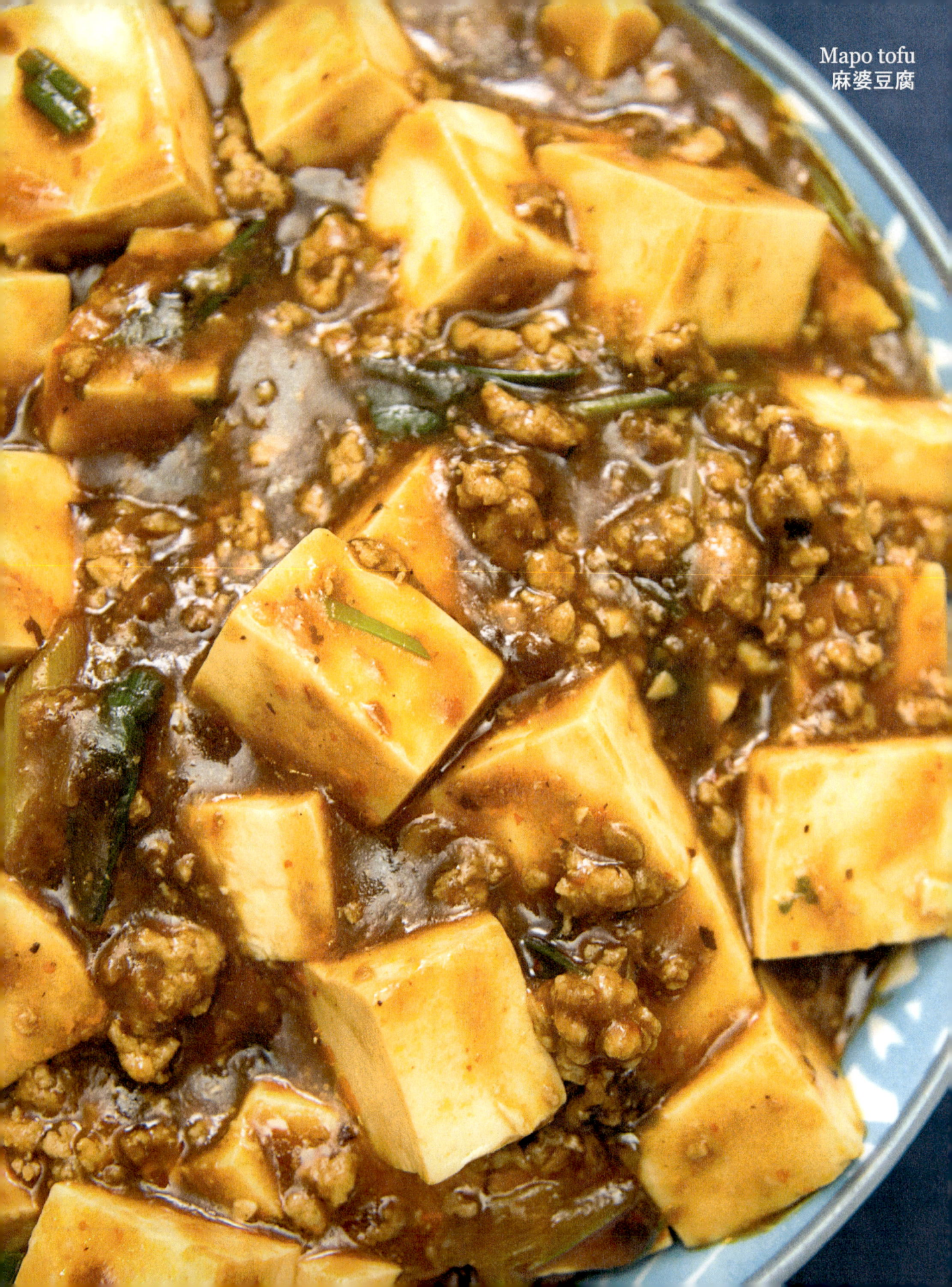

Mapo tofu
麻婆豆腐

Mapo-tofu 麻婆豆腐

Japanese style mapo-tofu is one of my favorite ways to enjoy tofu. It's extremely easy to make and not overly spicy. This is a classic Japanese style version of the famous Szechuan tofu dish.

SERVES 4-6

INGREDIENTS

2 blocks soft tofu
½ lb. ground pork
1 Tbsp garlic, crushed
1 Tbsp ginger, minced
2-3 green onions, sliced
2-3 Tbsp extra-virgin olive oil

For the sauce
2 Tbsp soy sauce
3 Tbsp tenmenjian
3 Tbsp tobanjian
2 Tbsp touchi (black bean paste)
1½ cups chicken stock

To thicken
4 tsps potato starch, dissolved in 2 Tbsp of water

DIRECTIONS

1. Cut the tofu into bite size pieces, measure out ingredients, and set aside.
2. Heat a large skillet on high heat. Add extra-virgin olive oil and pork, break into small pieces, and cook until slightly browned.
3. Add 2 Tbsp soy sauce with tenmenjian and add to pan with pork.
4. Next add ginger, garlic, tobanjian and mix a few times while cooking for 30-45 seconds.
5. Next, add in the chicken stock, black bean paste, and green onions and cook for 2-3 minutes mixing occasionally.
6. Add in the potato starch slurry and stir to incorporate. The sauce should thicken up noticeably within a minute.
7. Once the sauce has thickened, add the tofu and fold sauce into tofu.
8. Garnish with green onions and serve with rice +/- sansho pepper and la-yu.

Notes - Touchi (トウチ) – may be difficult to find, you can use Chinese black bean paste instead.
- If you can't find tenmenjian (甜麵醬), you can substitute by mixing 2 Tbsp miso, 1 tsp soy sauce, a pinch of sugar and drop of sesame oil. Mix together before combining with other ingredients.
- Tobanjian (豆板醬) has varying levels of spicyness. In my experience, Japanese versions tend to be more mild than Chinese brands. If you like your mapo-tofu spicy, be liberal with it and add a few extra teaspoons.
- For an additional layer of flavor/heat, consider adding some sansho pepper or red pepper flakes.

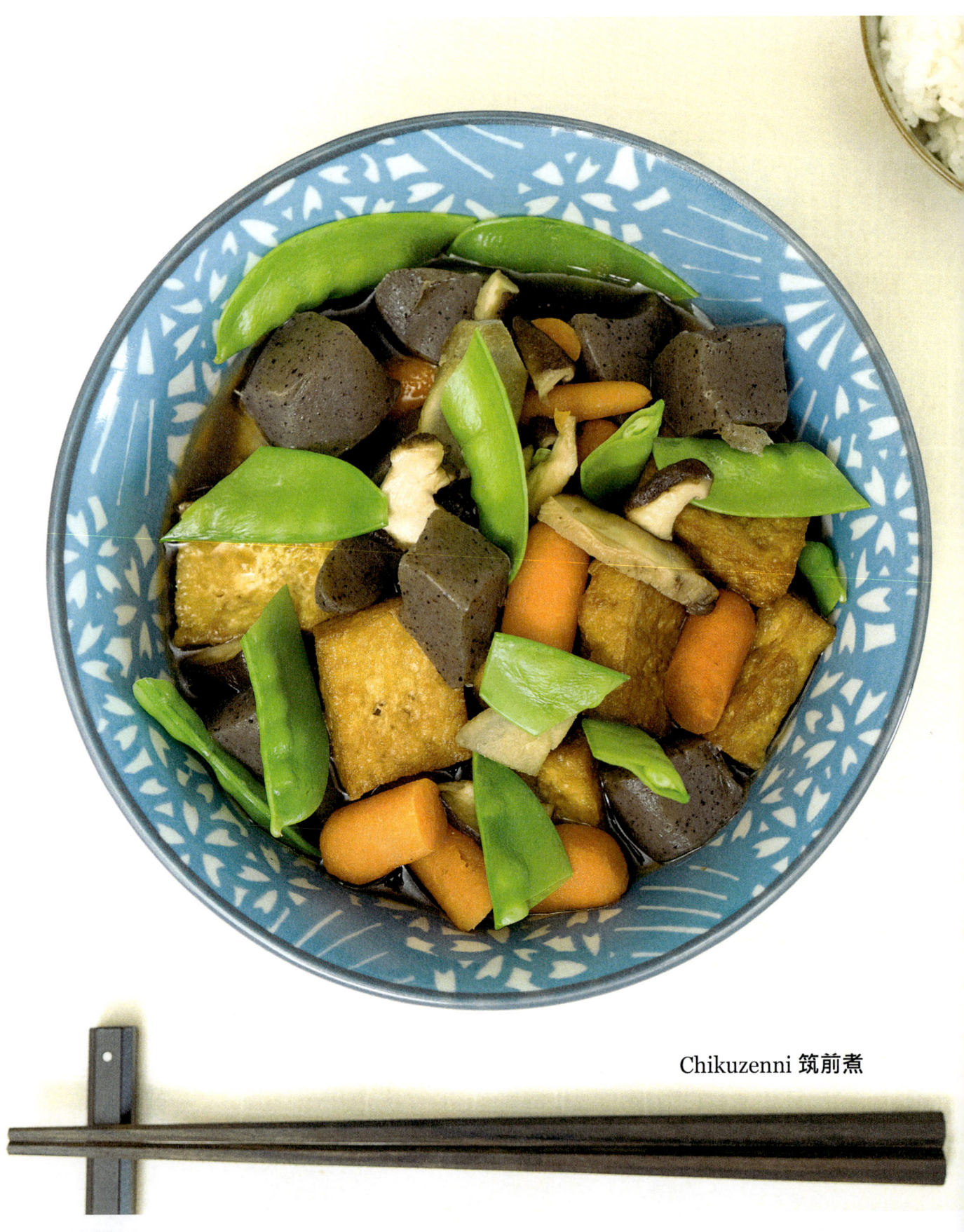

Chikuzenni 筑前煮

Chikuzenni 筑前煮

Chikuzenni is traditionally made with chicken and to celebrate New Year's. This variation is quite similar thanks to the firm texture of atsuage (deep fried tofu). Atsuage makes for an excellent substitute for chicken. It's got a firm outside texture and soft interior and can absorb the flavor of any sauce it's cooked in!

Serves 3-4

Ingredients

1½ cups atsuage cubes, *recipe P. 60*
1½ cups baby carrots
1 block konnyaku (8 oz), torn into cubes with a spoon
1 half piece gobo, (18 inches) deskinned and chopped
2-3 shiitake mushrooms, sliced
1 cup snow peas, microwaved for 30 seconds
1-2 Tbsp extra-virgin olive oil

For the broth
2 cups dashi, *recipe P. 23*
¼ cup sake
¼ cup mirin
¼ cup soy sauce
1 Tbsp sugar

Directions

1. Prepare your vegetables and tofu.
2. Measure out your sauce ingredients and set aside.
3. Use a small pot of boiling water to cook the konnyaku 2-3 minutes and drain liquid.
4. Add extra-virgin olive oil to a medium pot, add the carrots and gobo, cook on medium heat for 2-3 minutes.
5. Add in the dashi stock, shiitake mushrooms, konnyaku pieces, and simmer, partially covered for a minimum of 15-20 minutes. Cook up to 45+ minutes if you want soft vegetables or a more concentrated broth / completely dry dish.
6. Top with snow peas and serve with rice.

Tip - gobo (burdock root) may have a slight bitter flavor. If you're sensitive to it, try soaking in water after deskinning/cutting.
- Parboiling shirataki removes excess water and unpleasant flavor, allowing the simmering broth to penetrate.

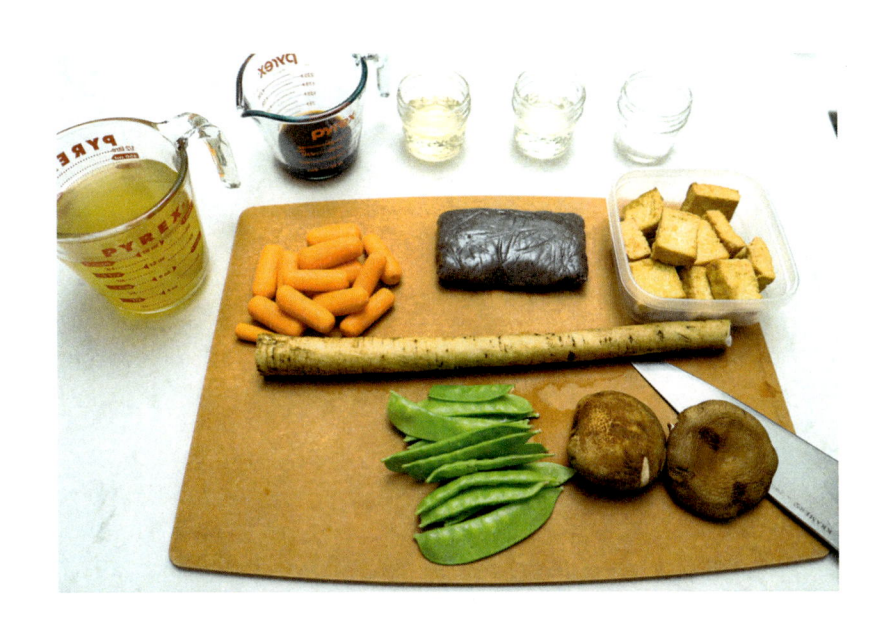

homemade soy milk

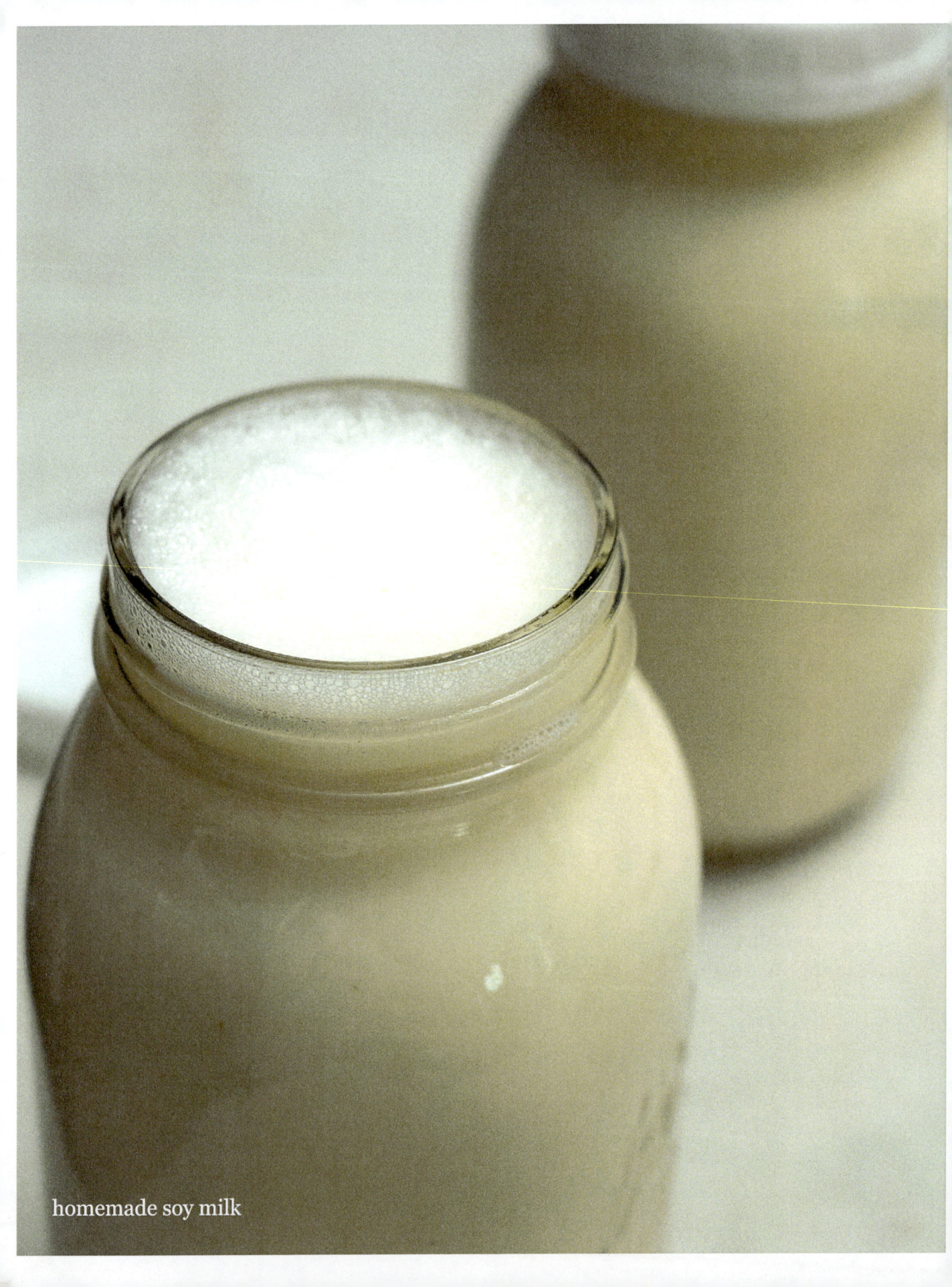

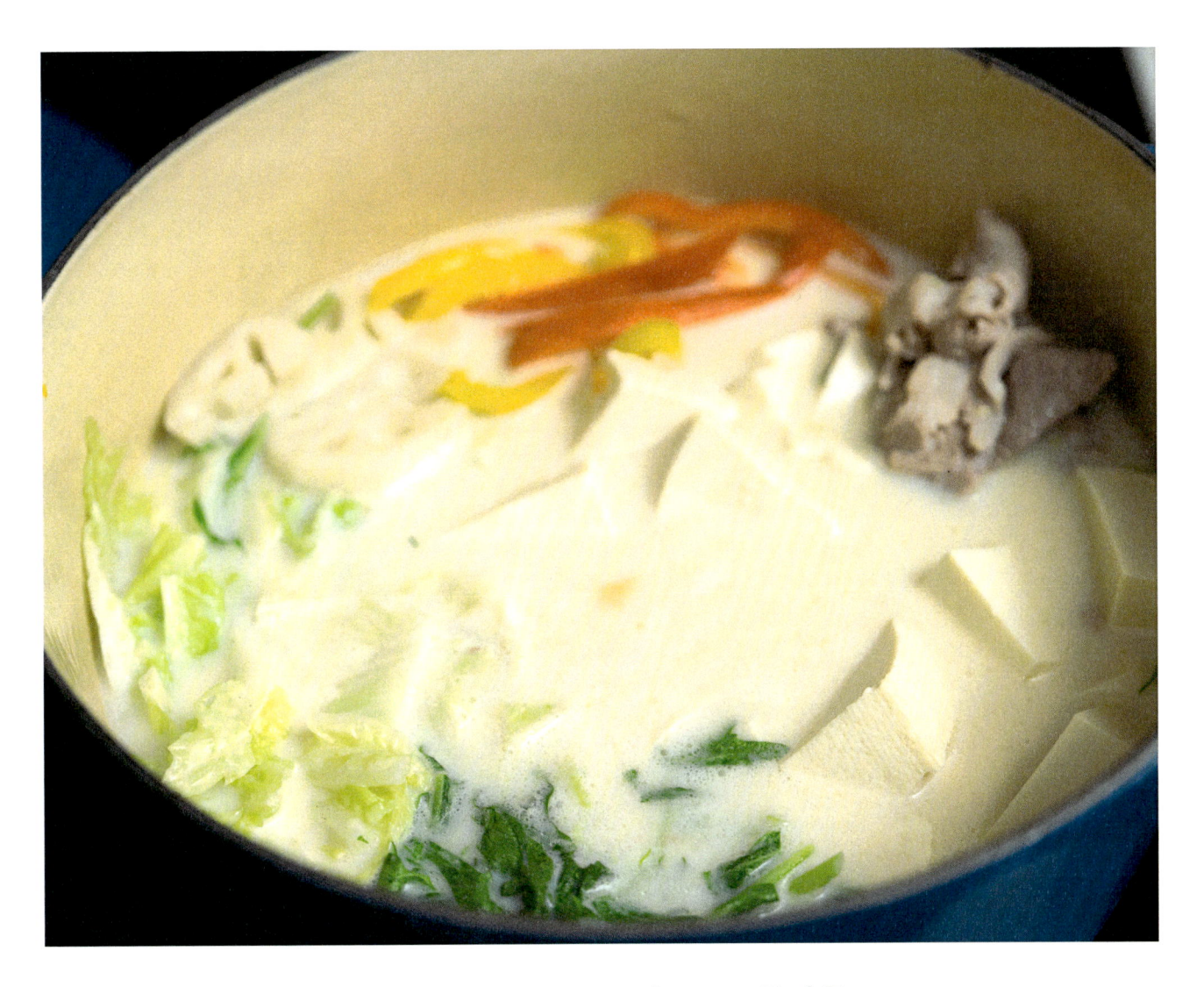

Tofu tounyuu nabe 豆腐豆乳鍋

Tounyuu nabe is a soy milk and konbu dashi based hot pot. It's delicate and creamy while at the same time providing just enough umami and flavor to complement a wide variety of ingredients.

It's one of my favorite ways to enjoy homemade tofu. The broth is very light and its mild flavor enables you to really enjoy the natural flavor of tofu.

If you can, I'd recommend using both homemade tofu and soy milk. Then you'll be experiencing this dish at it's full potential of flavor and tofu/soy deliciousness!

Just use the vegetables you have or that are in season and even leave out the meat!

Tofu has all the protein you need and the best part about this nabe? The variety of dipping sauces that'll keep you enjoying this for days and days!

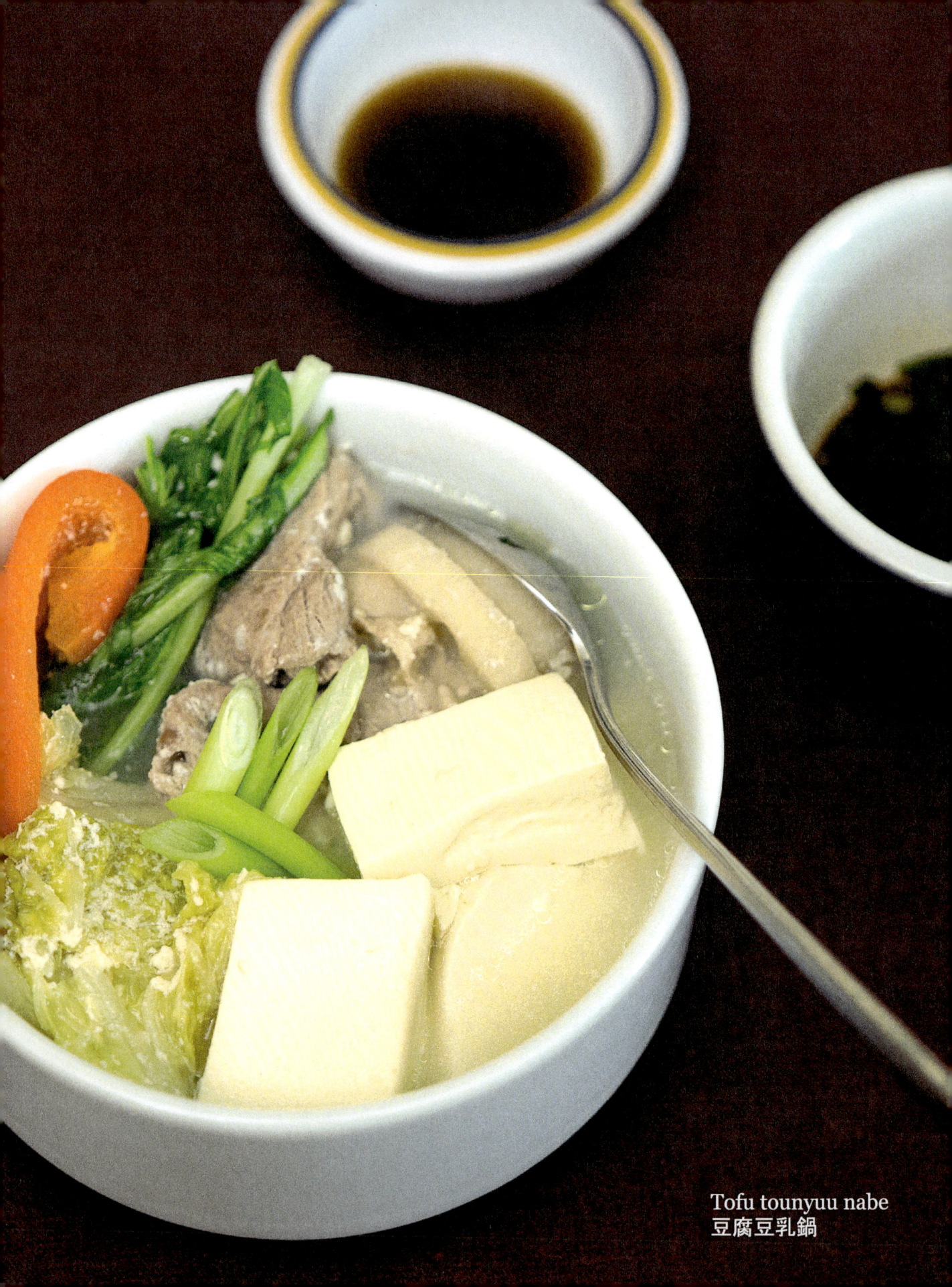

Tofu tounyuu nabe
豆腐豆乳鍋

Tofu tounyuu nabe 豆腐豆乳鍋

Use this as your base for a delicious hot pot with which you can serve a wide variety of toppings to keep you eating this all year long!

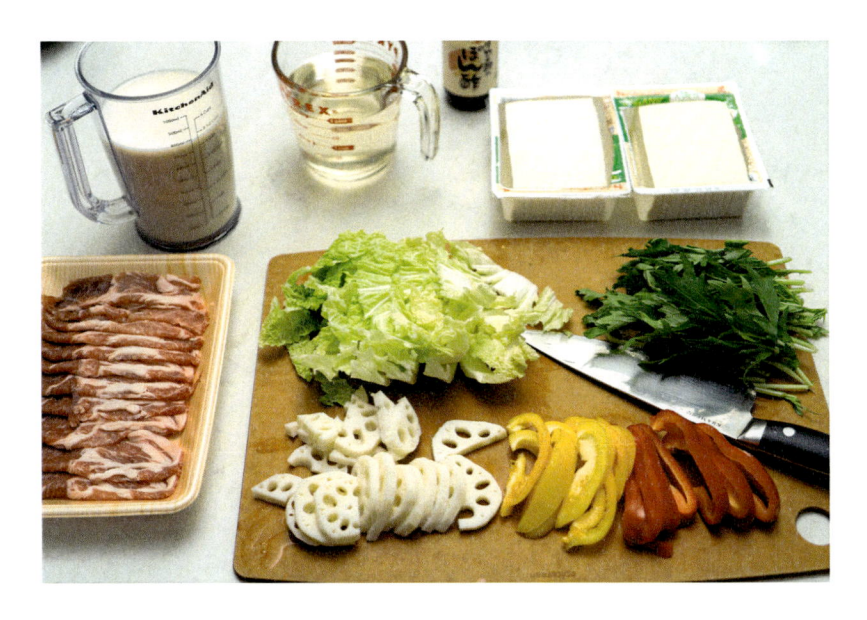

SERVES 4-6

Ingredients

2 blocks soft tofu
¼-½ lb. sliced pork
1½ cups renkon, peeled and sliced
½ red bell pepper
½ yellow bell pepper
2 cups napa cabbage
1½ cups mizuna or spinach
extra-virgin olive oil

Soup base
2 cups konbu dashi, recipe P. 21
3 cups soy milk

Optional- 1½ tsp baking soda (see tip)

Directions

1. Using a large dutch oven, cook pork in olive oil until slightly browned.
2. Meanwhile, prepare the vegetables. Slice renkon and bell peppers into ½ in. pieces, and cabbage/mizuna into 1-2 in. pieces.
3. Add all vegetables, soy milk and dashi to the dutch oven and bring to a simmer on medium heat.
4. Microwave tofu 2-3 minutes to remove excess water. Cut into bite size pieces and add to the pot.
5. Simmer on low heat for at least 15 minutes until heated through.
6. Serve with rice and dipping sauces on the following pages.

Tip - be careful not to use high heat as it will break down the soy milk and cause it to curdle and boil over.
- If using store-bought soy milk, stick with unflavored and unsweetened with minimal or no additives, if possible.
- If you're particular about the texture of your broth, consider adding in baking soda which decreases the pH of the broth and minimizes any curdling. Use 1/2 tsp per cup of soy milk.

Momiji oroshi
紅葉おろし

Momiji oroshi is a spicy and colorful way to add a kick to your daikon oroshi (大根おろし - grated daikon). The characters for momiji symbolize the leaves changing color in the Fall. Hence the name! Grated daikon is used to garnish many Japanese foods. So you can use this as a substitute if you're in the mood for something spicy!

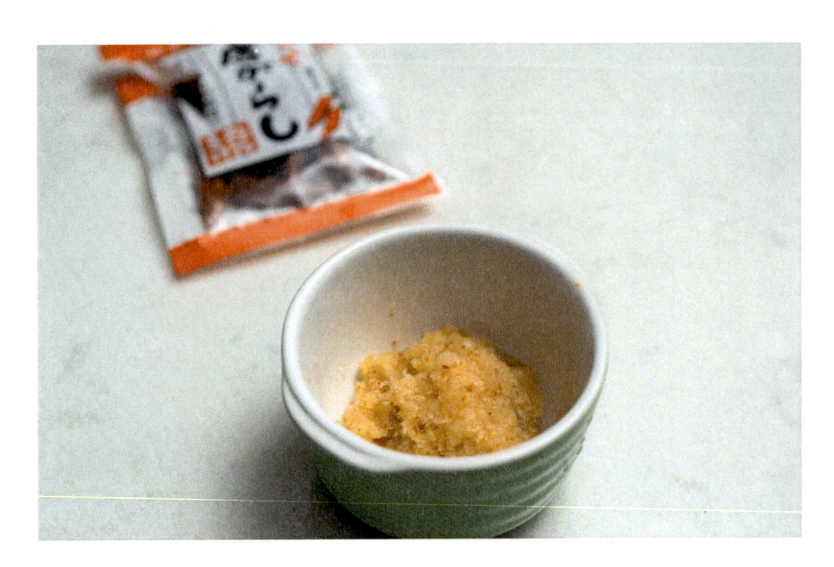

MAKES 1/4 CUP

INGREDIENTS

5-6 in. piece of daikon radish, peeled
3 dried red chiles, deseeded

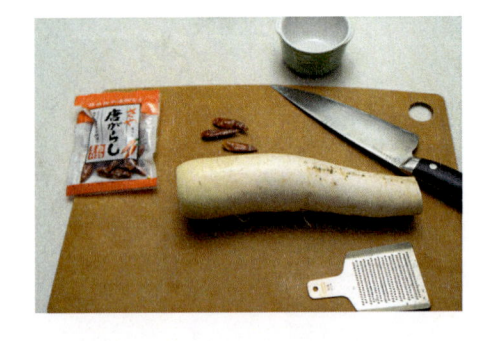

DIRECTIONS

1. Using a chopstick, make 3 holes near the center of one end of the daikon, approximately the depth of the longest red chile. Try to leave at least ½ in in between holes.
2. Deseed your red chiles by cutting into the side and scraping out. Use a little water if they don't come out all the way. Ensure you leave one end intact so that you can use it to push into the daikon.
3. Insert the dried chile into each hole and use a chopstick to push it down until flush with the surface.
4. Grate and strain excess water.
5. Serve as you would regular daikon oroshi - with fish, hiyayakko, nabemono (hot pot), hamburger or steak.

Tip- since chile is hot use a plastic bag to protect your skin or a fine mesh strainer if you don't want to get burned by the chile!

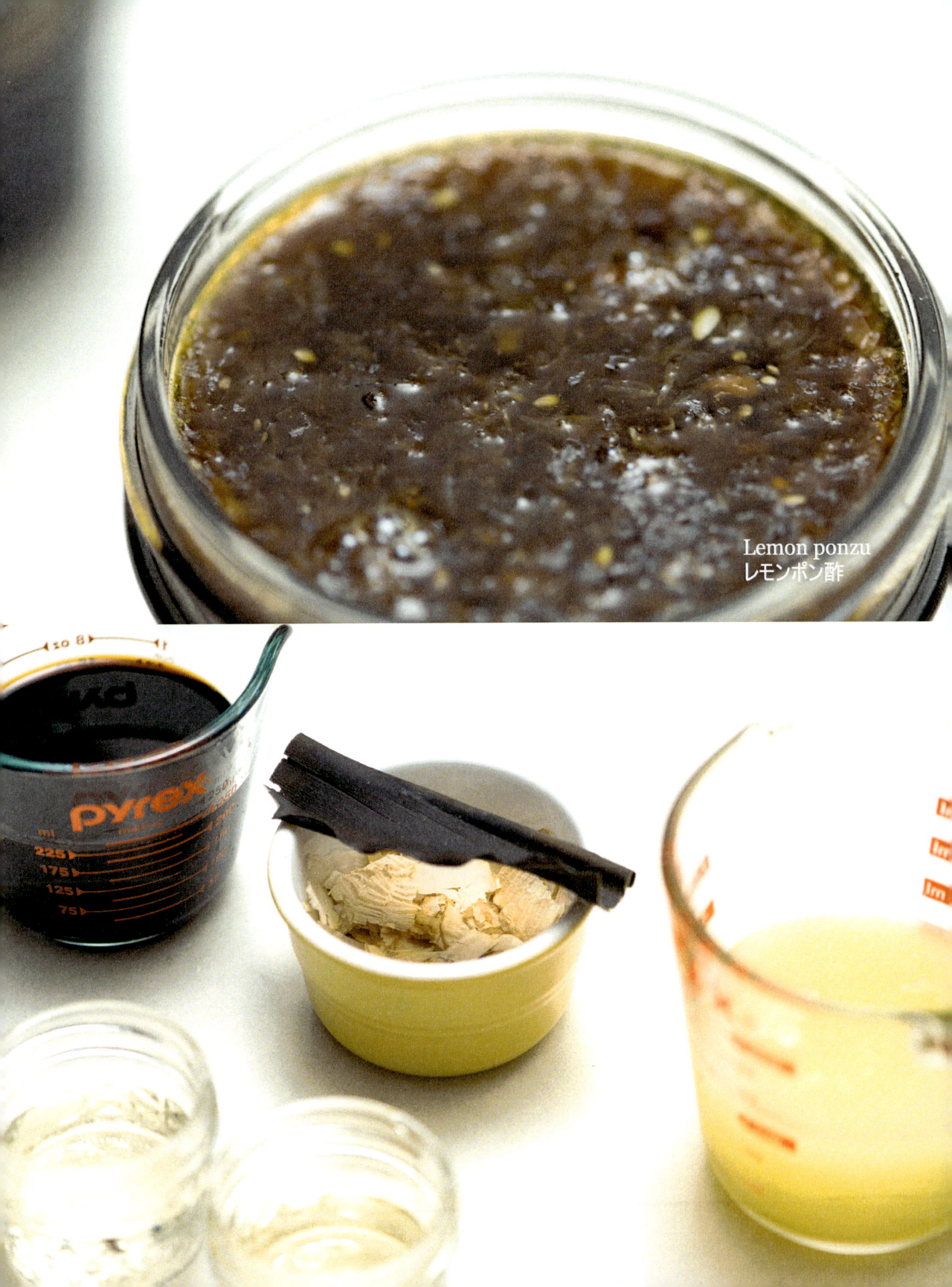

Lemon ponzu
レモンポン酢

Lemon ponzu レモンポン酢

Ponzu is a savory and tart sauce often made with citrus, soy sauce, and mirin. Though readily available at the store, there's nothing like making it from scratch. You can use this for many foods including gyoza, steamed vegetables, fish and more!

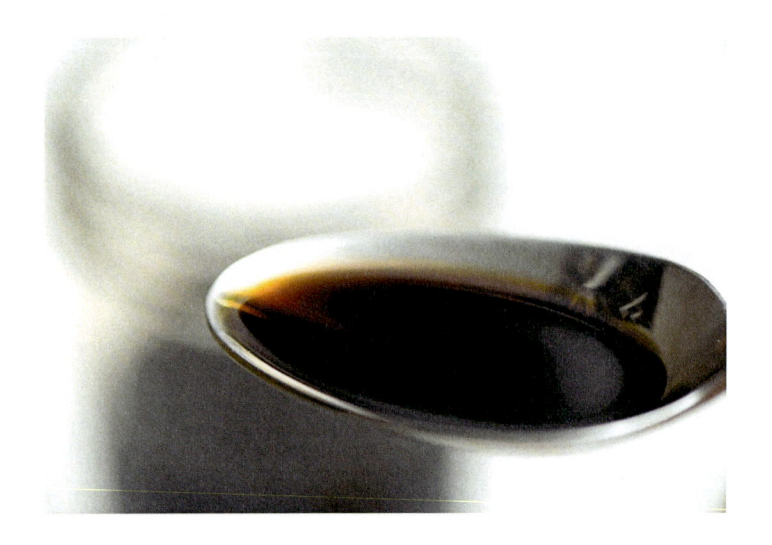

MAKES 2.5 CUPS

INGREDIENTS

1 cup soy sauce
1 cup lemon juice
¼ cup mirin
¼ cup sake
2-3 in. square piece of konbu (5g)
¼ cup katsuobushi flakes (5 g)

DIRECTIONS

1. Combine the mirin and sake in a small sauce pan and cook on medium heat until alcohol smell is gone, 2-3 minutes.
2. Add soy sauce and bring to just before a boil. Remove from heat and set aside.
3. In a large glass jar, add the lemon juice, konbu, and katsuobushi followed by the mirin, sake, and soy sauce mixture.
4. Store airtight in the refrigerator and wait at least 4-5 days before first use.
5. You can use this to season steamed vegetables, cooked fish, steak, sashimi (raw fish), and more!

Note- Use within 3-4 weeks. The flavor will develop gradually over time becoming more and more well-rounded.
- If you want a little more texture in your ponzu, save the pulp and add it with the juice.

Nirajouyu ニラ醤油

Nirajouyu is simply nira and soy sauce. However, I like to add in a little sake or mirin to enhance the flavor. Compared to sake, mirin adds a little more sweetness to round things out. Like ponzu, you can use this to season a wide variety of foods!

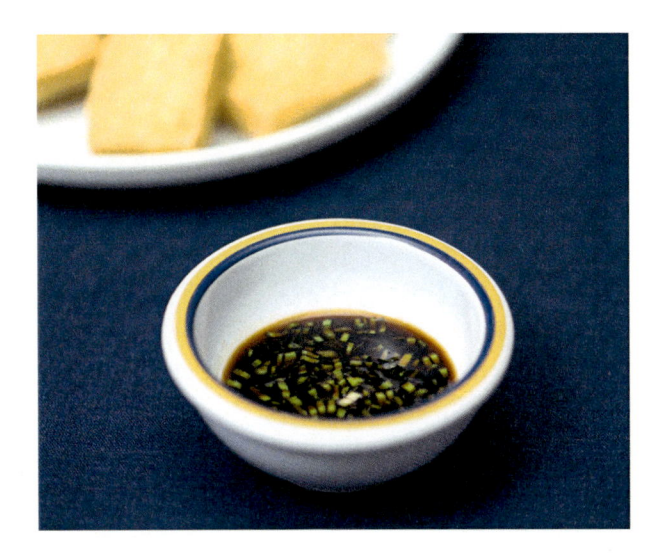

MAKES 1/4 CUP

INGREDIENTS

⅓ cup soy sauce
2 Tbsp mirin
2-3 Tbsp nira (garlic chives)

optional-
1 Tbsp sesame oil or crushed sesame seeds
red pepper flakes

DIRECTIONS

1. Microwave the mirin for about 30 seconds until the alcohol is gone.
2. Finely chop the nira and combine with soy sauce and mirin.
3. Serve with atsuage (*recipe P. 60*), tounyuu nabe (*recipe P. 85*), gyoza (*recipe P. 94*), steak, and fish!
4. Store airtight in the refrigerator and use within 2-3 days.

Note- Mirin with the alcohol cooked off is called (煮きりみりん - nikirimirin). Sake if cooked in the same way, is called nikirizake (煮きり酒). By cooking off the alcohol, you remove the sharp/bitter alcohol flavors and concentrate the naturally occurring umami compounds.

This technique can be used for other sauces/dishes where you want the umami mirin and sake provide, but are not cooking it. Examples include 'tare' for sushi, aemono (seasoned vegetables), and sunomono (pickled vegetables). Try it and see if you can notice the difference in flavor :)

Tofu hamburger
豆腐ハンバーグ

Hannbaagu (said with a Japanese accent) is generally a beef or pork patty, sometimes mixed with vegetables like onion, carrots, or renkon. When I'm in a meaty mood I'll use all meat, but when I'm looking for lighter fare, I'll use chicken with tofu!

SERVES 4

INGREDIENTS

½ lb. firm tofu
½ lb. ground chicken or pork
1-2 cloves garlic, crushed
½ cup onion, chopped
dash of salt and black pepper
dash of nutmeg
½ tsp chicken stock paste
1 egg
¾ cup panko
2-3 Tbsp extra-virgin olive oil

For the Sauce
¼ cup ketchup
2 Tbsp chuno or Worcestershire sauce
2 Tbsp sake
2 Tbsp mirin
2 Tbsp butter

DIRECTIONS

1. Microwave tofu in a paper towel lined bowl for 2 minutes. Meanwhile, chop the onion.
2. When tofu is done, remove and allow to cool. Microwave onions for at least 2 minutes while you prepare the other ingredients.
3. Using a large bowl combine the chicken, panko, garlic, chicken stock paste, salt, black pepper, and nutmeg. Then add tofu, onion, and mix thoroughly.
4. Shape into the patties about ½ in. thick and 3-4 in. in diameter. Set aside.
5. Heat 2-3 Tbsp extra-virgin olive oil on a large pan using medium heat. Once heated, add patties and cook until slightly browned and flip.
6. Once flipped, add in 1-2 Tbsp water to steam and cover with a lid to expedite cooking. Repeat for the remaining patties.
7. Once cooked, place on serving plate, top with sauce.
8. Serve with steamed vegetables, potatoes and/or rice.

For the sauce
1. Mix together all ingredients in a saucepan and heat on medium heat. Stir continuously and cook for 5-7 minutes.
2. Once the alcohol smell is gone, remove from heat and set aside.

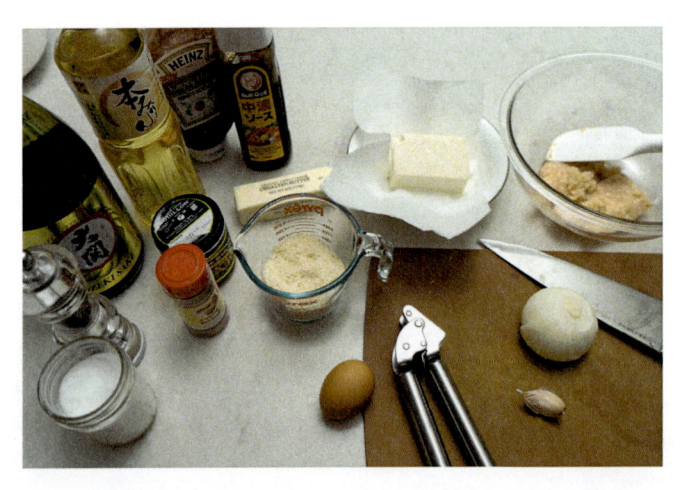

Tofu hamburger 豆腐ハンバーグ

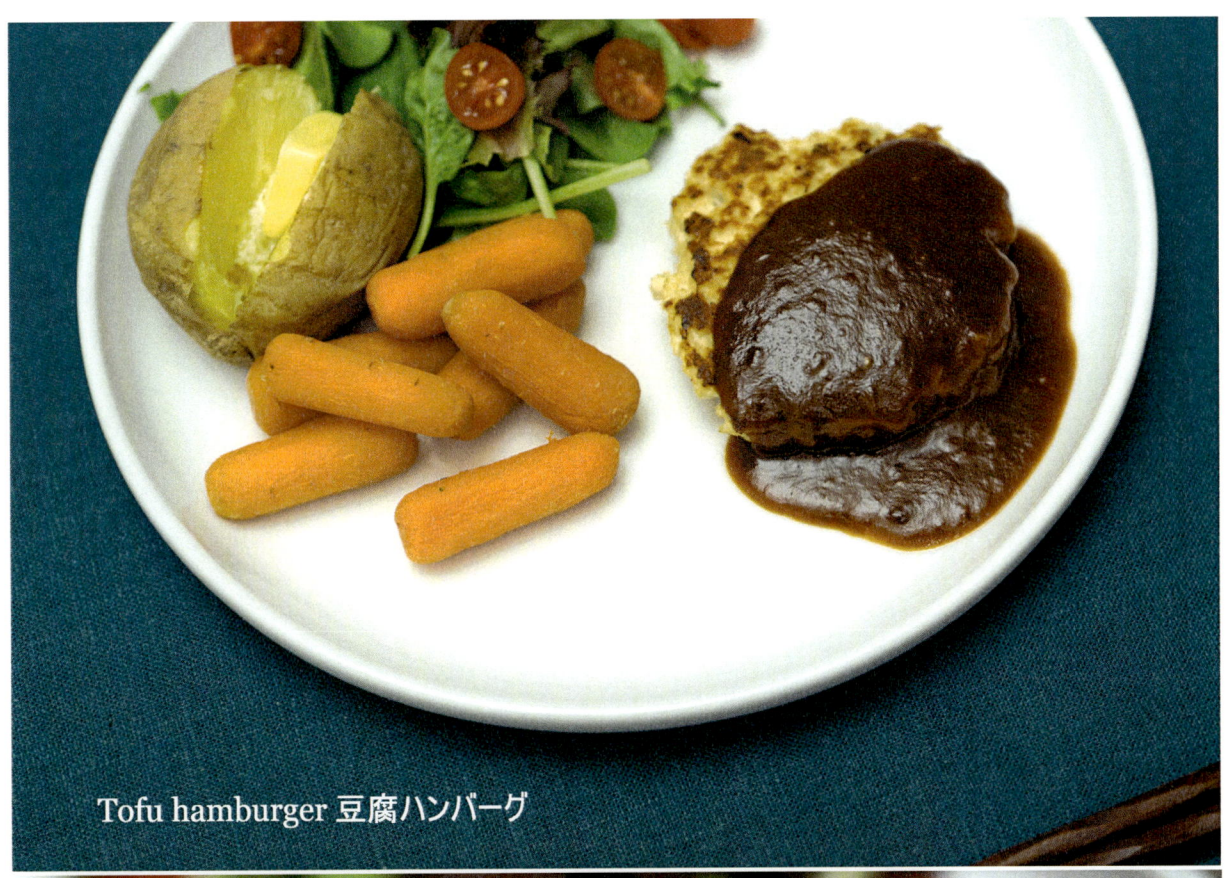

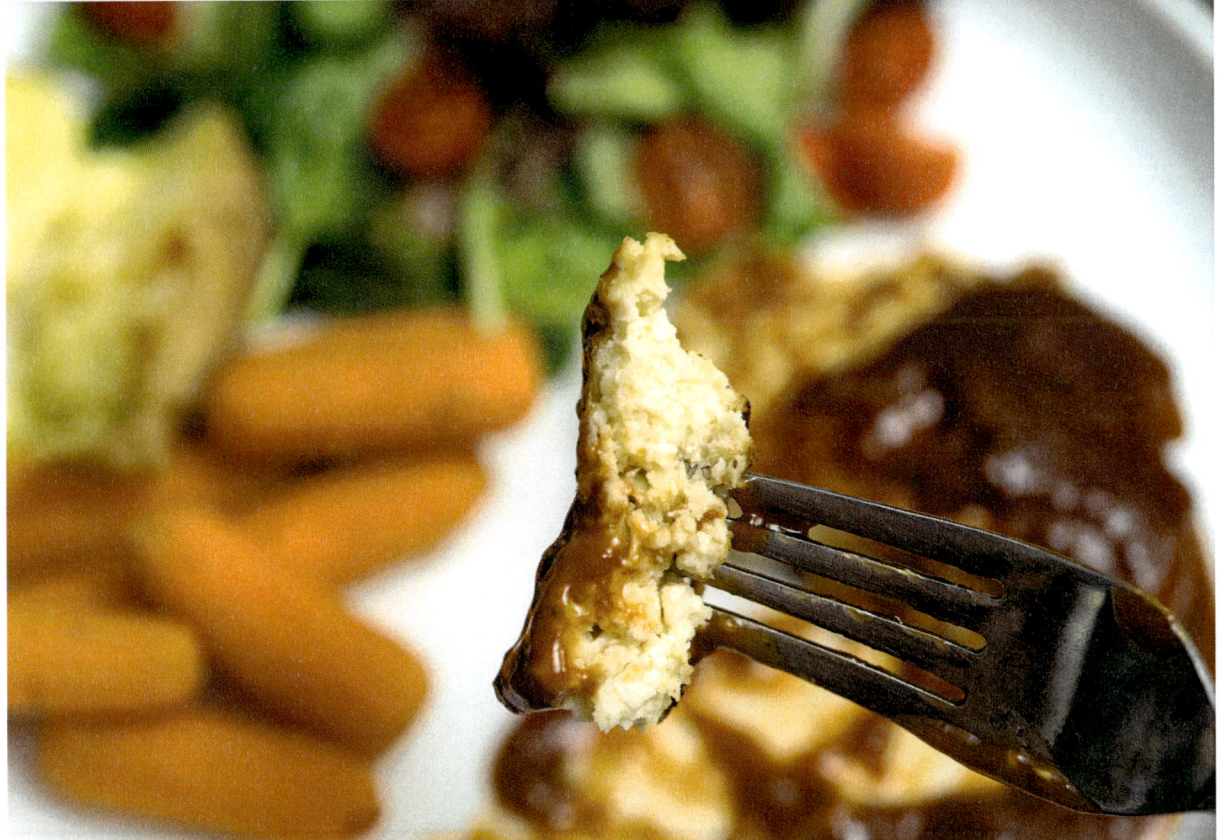

Nikudoufu 肉豆腐

If you love sukiyaki, you'll love nikudoufu. Never had it? Both are wonderfully rich, simmered foods seasoned with soy sauce, mirin, and sake. Japanese comfort food at it's best! Mushrooms and snow peas are a delicious way to add some vegetables to this hearty and classic meat and tofu dish.

SERVES 4

Ingredients

2 blocks firm tofu, cut into ½ in. rectangles
1 package shirataki noodles (14 oz)
½ lb. sliced beef
1 white onion, sliced
2-4 shiitake mushrooms, sliced
½ bunch enoki mushrooms
1 cup snow peas or 1 stalk green onion, chopped

For the broth
1 cup mirin
½ cup water
½ cup sake
½ cup soy sauce
2-3 in. square piece of konbu (5g)
1 Tbsp sugar

Directions

1. Prepare your vegetables and tofu.
2. Use a large saute pan and lightly pan fry your tofu pieces in 2-3 Tbsp extra-virgin olive oil. This helps to add a nice texture.
3. Measure out all broth ingredients and set aside.
4. Use a small pot of boiling water to cook the shirataki 2-3 minutes. Remove from the pot and use the same water to cook the beef 2-3 minutes. Drain cooking liquids.
5. Cut the shirataki noodles once or twice with scissors or a knife.
6. Add all ingredients including broth to a large pot. Simmer partially covered for at least 15-20 minutes.
7. Meanwhile, microwave snow peas for a minute and set aside.
7. Once the nikudoufu has cooked, serve with rice and top with snow peas or chopped green onion.

Tips - if you are sensitive to spicy onions, after slicing allow to soak in cold water for 5 to 10 minutes. Any longer and you'll lose the onion flavor. Pat dry before adding to the pot.
- Parboiling shirataki removes excess water and unpleasant flavor, allowing the simmering broth to be better absorbed by the noodles.
- Parboiling the beef removes scum and some fat, which results in a cleaner flavor.
- A lower-calorie alternative to pan-frying your tofu is broiling for a few minutes in the oven.

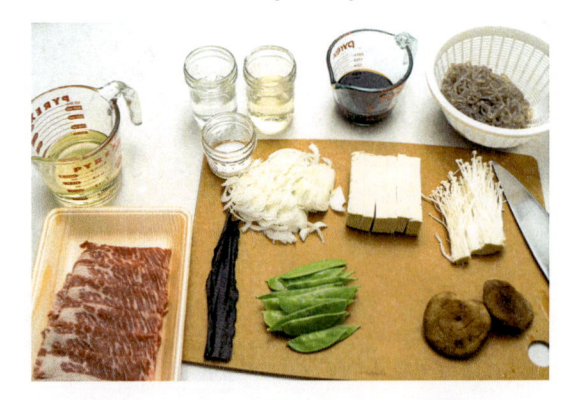

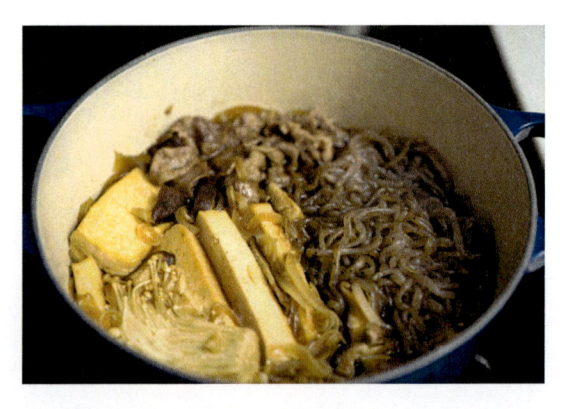

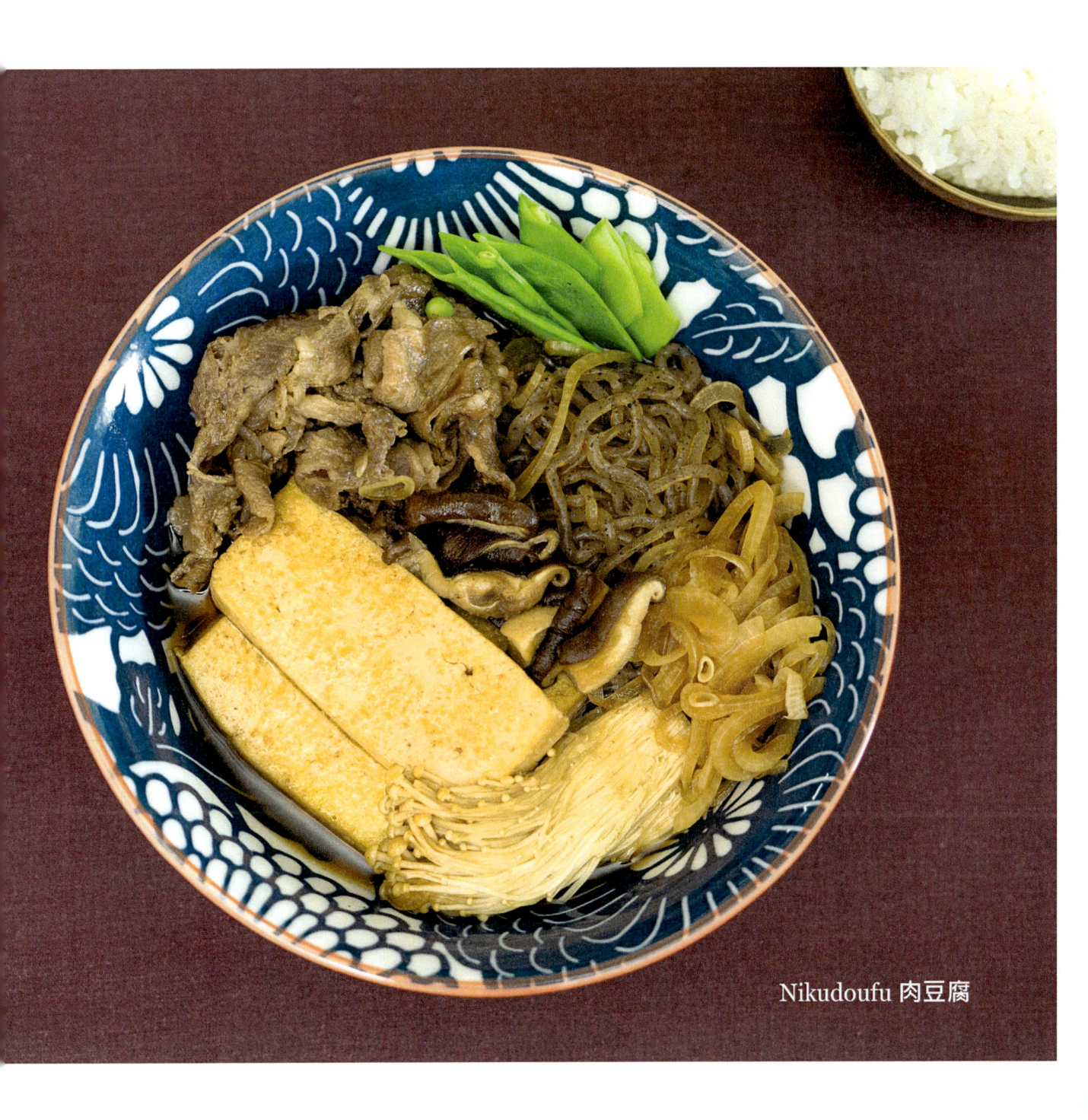

Nikudoufu 肉豆腐

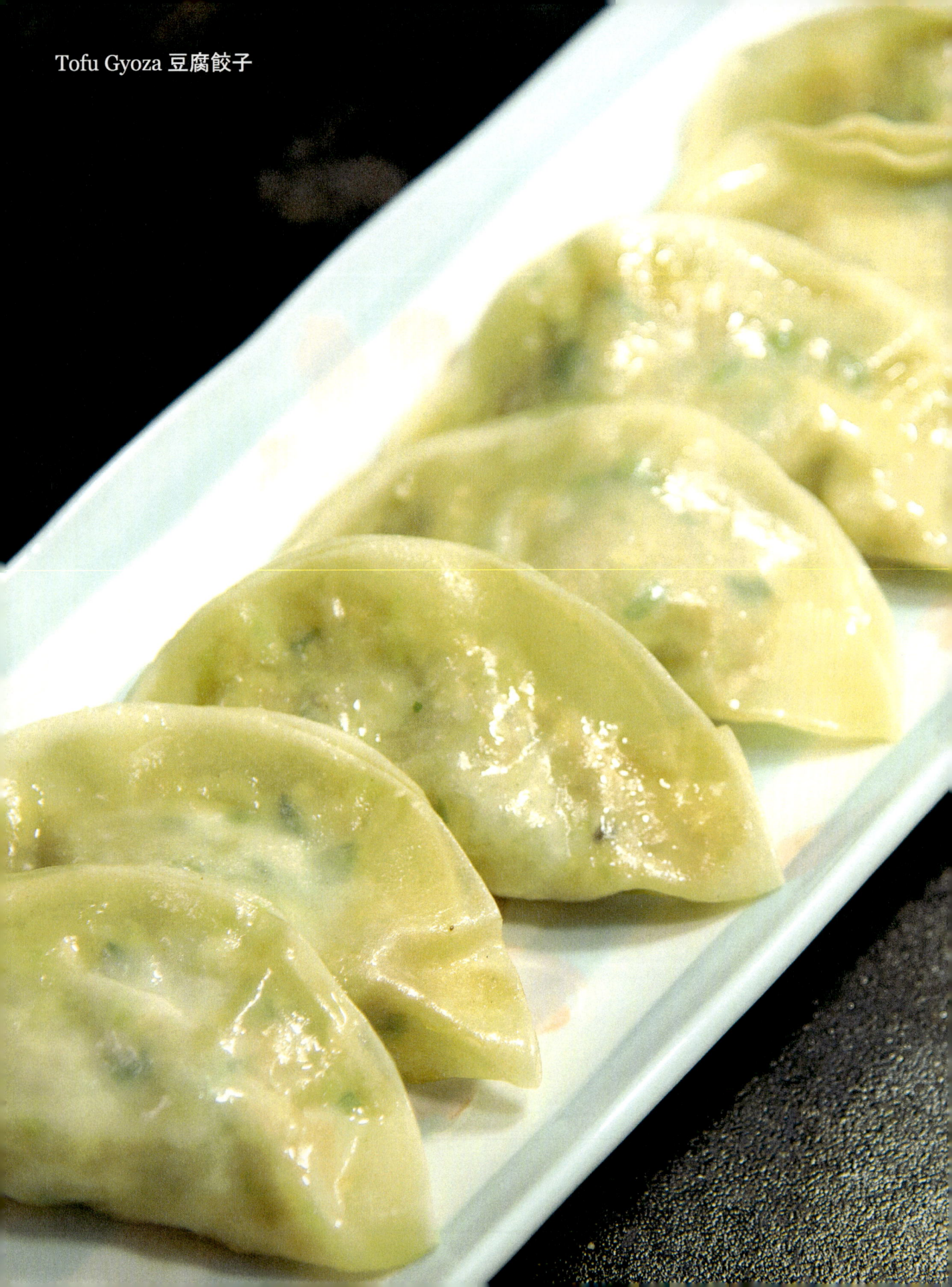

Tofu Gyoza 豆腐餃子

Tofu gyoza 豆腐餃子

There's nothing like piping hot gyoza! Crunchy on the outside and full of delicious goodness on the inside. These gyoza have a little extra bite on the inside thanks to the moyashi (bean sprouts), while tofu and nira serve as the perfect filler for a meatless meal.

SERVES 4

INGREDIENTS

1 block firm tofu
2 ½ cups bean sprouts (200 grams), finely chopped)
2 Tbsp soy sauce
2 Tbsp potato starch
1 tsp dashi powder
1 Tbsp ginger
1 Tbsp garlic, crushed
2-3 Tbsp nira (garlic chives), finely chopped
white pepper
4-6 Tbsp extra-virgin olive oil for pan-frying

30-50 Gyoza skins
Small bowl of water for dipping fingers

For serving
Rice vinegar, soy sauce,

DIRECTIONS

1. Use your hands or a firm spatula to break tofu into little pieces, roughly 1/4 in. for the thickest pieces.
2. Combine with bean sprouts, soy sauce, potato starch, dashi powder, ginger, garlic, nira, and white pepper. Mix thoroughly
3. Prepare a large plate or baking sheet covered with parchment for your folded gyoza.
4. To make each gyoza, add 2-3 teaspoons of the filling to a gyoza wrapper, dip your finger in water, paint one edge of the wrapper, and fold in half.
5. If you wish to crease your skins, fold the side facing away from you against itself, while holding one end in place. Repeat to create 3-5 folds.
6. Heat a large cast iron pan with oil. Once shimmering, add gyoza and cook about 1-2 minutes until the bottom develops a nice brown crust or kitsuneiro (the color of a fox, in Japanese - きつね色).
7. At this point, you'll need to rotate or turn each piece on its side or it may burn.
8. To steam, carefully add a few tablespoons of water to the pan and cover immediately. Cook for another 2-3 minutes, until heated through. This will give you gyoza that are both soft and crunchy with each bite.
9. Serve with rice along with La-yu, rice vinegar and soy sauce.

*IMPORTANT - thoroughly remove excess water from the tofu. Also, pat dry your moyashi after rinsing! Too much water left = soggy and broken wrappers.
- For extra crispy gyoza, just use oil without the steaming method above.
- Be careful when adding water as it will splatter with the oil. Immediately cover with a lid and cook for another 30-45 seconds to steam.
- Use a flat spatula or fish spatula to remove from the pan to prevent breaking the skins of the cooked gyoza.*

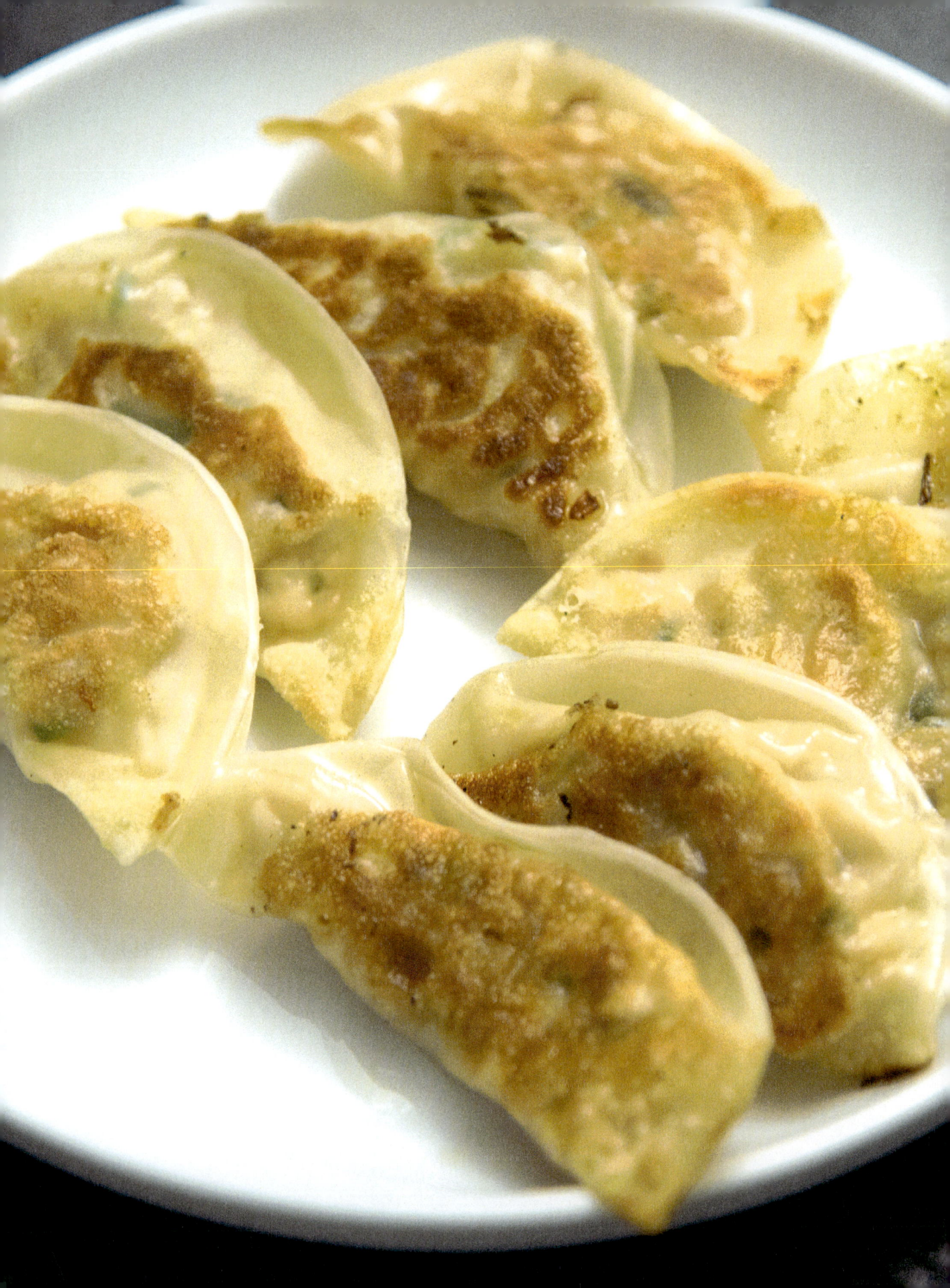

Shimantogawa River, Kochi Prefecture, Japan

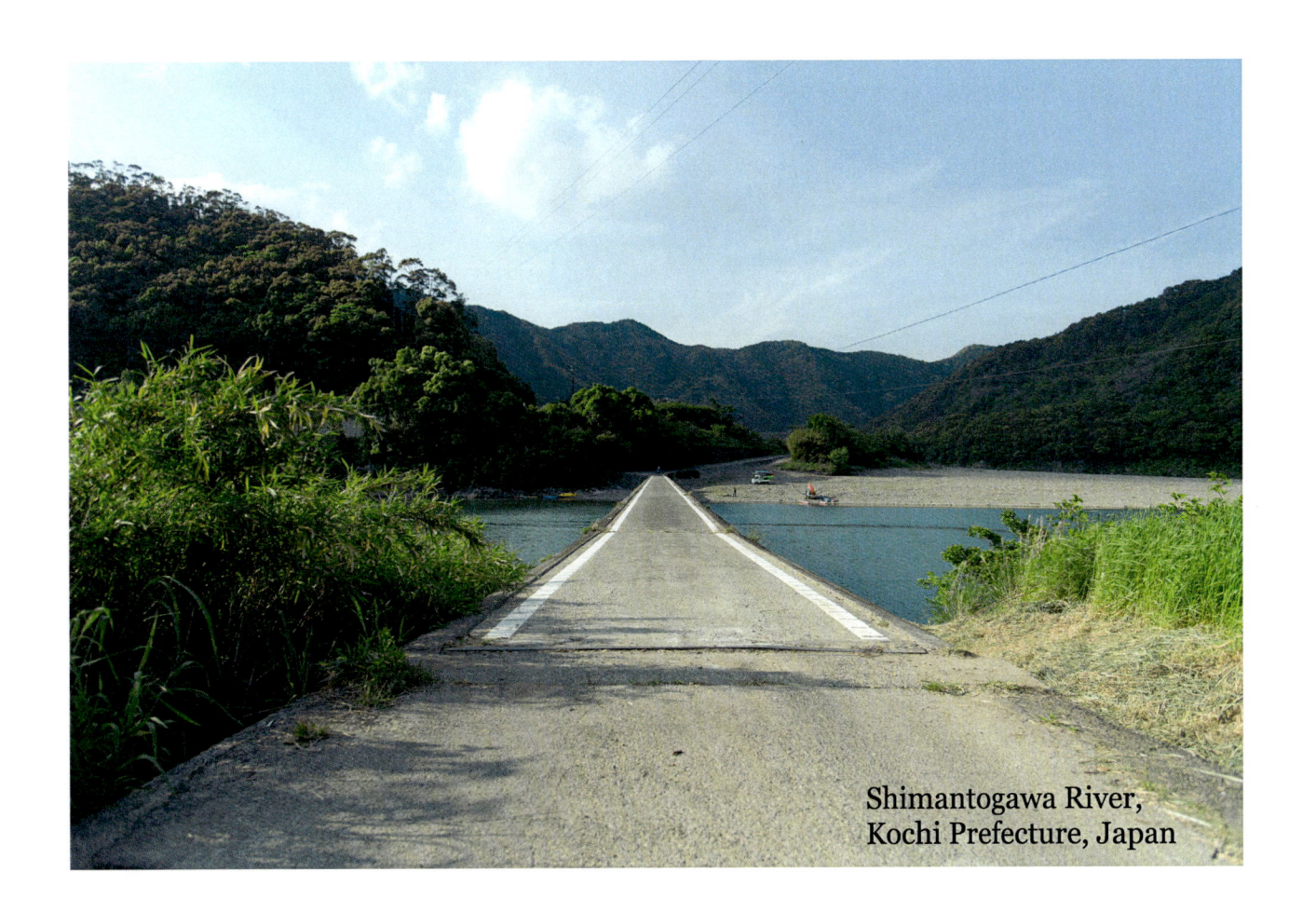

Next Steps

Learning doesn't stop with this book. Make sure to get your FREE bonus materials at www.alldayieat.com/bookbonus

If you have any questions or comments, please email me at patrick@alldayieat.com

Share your recreations and tag me on Facebook @alldayieat or Instagram @alldayieatlikeashark #alldayieat #tofuryouri

Subscribe to my Youtube channel for weekly Japanese cooking videos!

Thank you for buying this book!

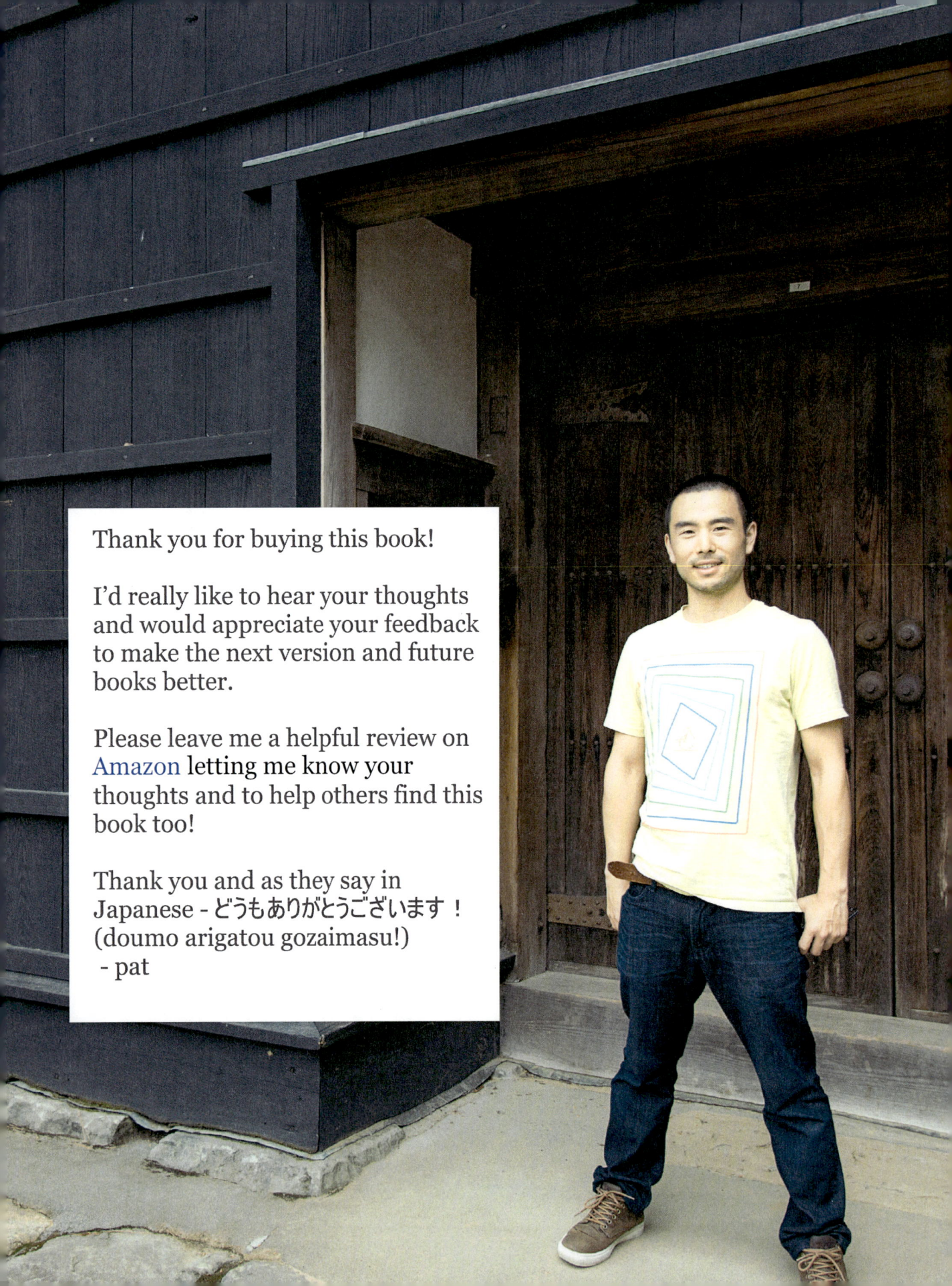

I'd really like to hear your thoughts and would appreciate your feedback to make the next version and future books better.

Please leave me a helpful review on Amazon letting me know your thoughts and to help others find this book too!

Thank you and as they say in Japanese - どうもありがとうございます！
(doumo arigatou gozaimasu!)
 - pat

About the Author

When Pat was a kid he hated eating sushi, but loved Big Macs with a large order of fries. As he grew older, his tastes matured and he embarked on a seemingly never ending journey around the world just to eat. One day his dream is to take a big trip with his girlfriend to travel the world. One more time. They traveled around Asia for 6 months in 2012. On that trip they bought a pair of darumasan. When they came back they painted one eye of the darumasan to wish for the opportunity to take another big trip to continue exploring the world. Perhaps by 2020 he says. At which point, they'll draw in the other eye of the darumasan. He lives in Orange County, California and when not cooking and eating, he likes to roast coffee, surf, and enjoy live music.

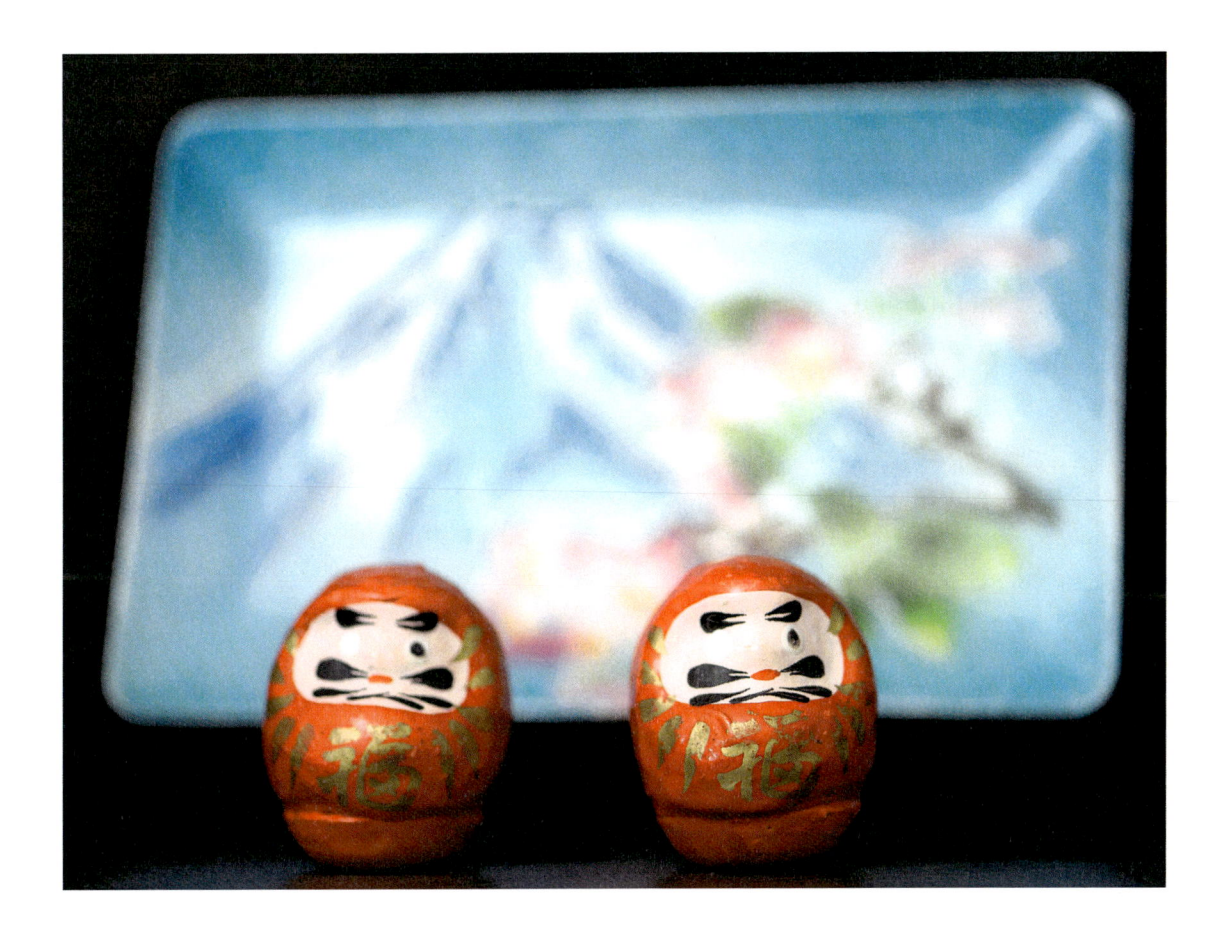

Acknowledgements

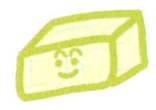

A big thank you to the people who have helped support and make this book possible -

Jonathan Chambers - owner of Laurasoybeans.com, an excellent place to get your soybeans for soy milk, tofu, and all the other tasty products of soy!

Namiko Chen - the creator of JustOneCookbook.com, a site that's focused on Japanese cuisine with an entire library of Japanese recipes, videos, and more!

Sarah Hodge - a Japan-based food and travel writer for several publications including Tokyo Weekender and Stars and Stripes Japan. She has a strong interest in Shojin ryouri.

Emi Minejima - my partner in crime who taste-tested many pounds of tofu and helped me figure out what could be improved.

Roberta Schwartz - a registered nurse based in Maryland, who has a keen interest in gardening, cooking, and Japanese cuisine and culture.

Tommy Alderman - one half of the Alderman Farms operation, who being the excellent homesteader he is, planted a few seeds that helped me on my path to this book!

My parents - who have always been supportive of my projects and helped to guide me in countless ways on my journey through life.

My previous All day I Eat Japanese food students. All of whom not only share a passion for cooking and eating, but were also gracious and patient with me as I launched and tested several online Japanese cooking courses. You guys know I wouldn't be where I am today without your feedback and support!

Class of 2018
Louisa M.
Mary W.
Danielle K.
Dezer K.
Enna R.
Eugene S.
Jessica M.
Kristina D.
Cat L.
Michael V.
Sam P.
Tim S.
Marie-Laure A.
Marianna S.
Hasybi R.
Maria A.
Henry B.
Eric R.
Pamela M.
Naomi S.
Meriko F.
Alice K.

Class of 2017
Valerie S.
Sharon S.
Patti W.
Nicole B.
Hazel G.
Jonathan L.
Shaun O.
Kira K.
Lewis P.
Robin S.

Resources

For books on food, Japanese pantry ingredients, cookware, and more - visit
www.alldayieat.com/resources

For more Japanese recipes and cooking videos visit www.alldayieat.com

Get your FREE bonus materials at www.alldayieat.com/bookbonus

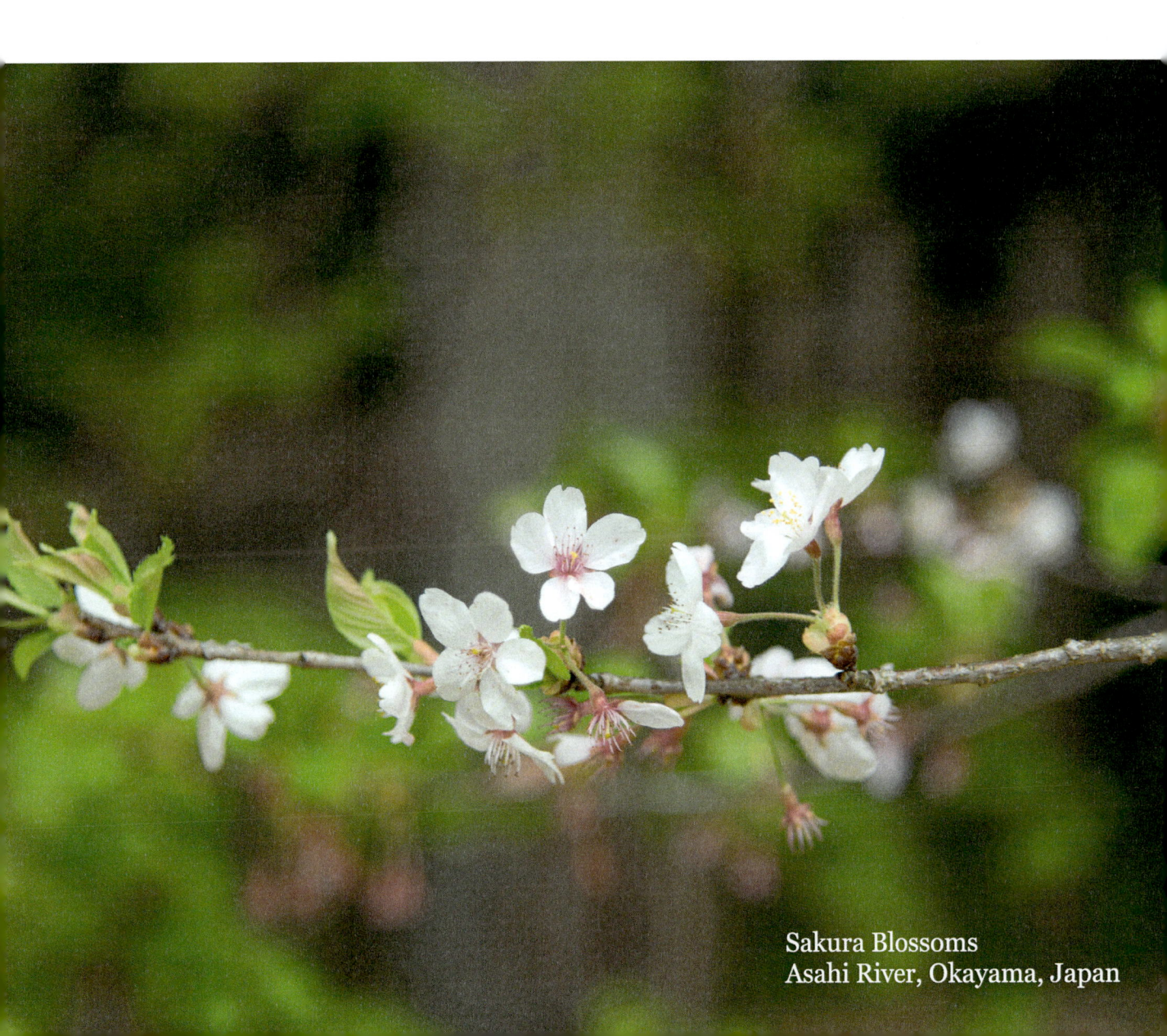

Sakura Blossoms
Asahi River, Okayama, Japan

Frequently Asked Questions

How long will tofu keep once opened?

I recommend you use your tofu within 2-3 days of opening the package. If you don't use it right away make sure to cover airtight and store in the refrigerator. If you leave it uncovered you'll dry out the surface and it may develop an unpleasant sliminess. Some people say to store in water and change it out daily, but I usually store without water and it works just fine.

Can I freeze tofu?

Yes, **but** you'll ruin the texture. **A big but** there. Once defrosted it'll be a watery and spongy mess. For the recipes in this book this is not recommended!

Why is there water in the tofu package?

This helps to minimize the tofu from breaking and add a little bit of cushion for transport. Throw this away since there isn't much flavor or nutrition in it.

Why is my tofu water yellow?

The natural pigment from the tofu may have leaked into the water, if it tastes or smells funny either because it's not fresh (past expiration) or you opened it several days ago... toss it.

How to best enjoy tofu?

As tofu is an already cooked product, you don't need to recook it. You can eat it straight out of the container. However, cooking with tofu does give you some more options on seasoning and is one of my favorite ways of enjoying it.

How to cook tofu?

Tofu is extremely versatile. You can do just about anything with it, sauté, boil, fry, grill, bake, steam, or even microwave it. Hopefully, some of the recipes in this book will inspire you to cook more tofu and think of new ways to enjoy it!

Made in the USA
San Bernardino, CA
18 January 2019